FASTING DIET FOR

BEGINNERS

KETO DIETS AND INTERMITTENT FASTING

GUIDE TO KETO DIETS AND INTERMITTENT FASTING

CONTENTS

ABOUT THE BOOK

Starting the ketogenic diet and intermittent fasting can be overwhelming, so much to learn, so many resources to choose from. So why doesn't somebody make it easy? We did. This Complete Ketogenic Diet and intermittent fasting guide for Beginners is your all-in-one resource for starting and sticking to the ketogenic diet. You get exactly what you need to make keto surprisingly simple; meal plans, shopping lists, support, and lots of keto recipes.

For too long we've blamed dietary fat for weight gain and health problems. The truth is, a diet that's high in natural, healthy fats can actually help your body burn fat! That's the secret behind the ketogenic diet. As you get more of your calories from healthy fats and cut back on carbs, you'll start burning fat, losing weight, and feeling strong and energetic.

The Keto Diet does away with the "one size fits all" philosophy offering a customizable approach that is tailored to the unique needs of the individual.

A one-stop guide to the ketogenic way of eating, The Keto Diet shows you how to transition to and maintain a whole foods-based, paleo-friendly, ketogenic diet with a key focus on practical strategies - and tons of mouthwatering recipes.

INTRODUCTION

The ketogenic diet has become popular as a therapy for epilepsy in the 1920s and 1930s. It was developed to provide an alternative to the non-mainstream fasting, which had demonstrated success as an epilepsy therapy. However, the diet was eventually largely abandoned due to the introduction of new anticonvulsive therapies. Although it emerged that most cases of epilepsy could be effectively managed using these medications, they still did not achieve epilepsy control in around 20% 30% of epileptics. For these individuals, and particularly children with epilepsy, the diet was reintroduced as a technique to control the condition.

The role of fasting in the treatment of disease has been known to mankind for thousands of years and has been studied in detail by ancient Greek physicians and ancient Indian physicians. An early treatise on the Hippocratic corpus, "On Sacred Disease," describes how changes in diet played a role in the management of epilepsy.

The first modern scientific study on fasting as a cure for epilepsy was conducted in France in 1911. So potassium bromide was used to treat epilepsy, but this agent slowed patients' mental capacities. Instead, twenty patients of epilepsy followed a low-calorie, vegetarian food plan that was combined with fasting. Two patients showed significant improvements, although most could not adhere to dietary limitations. However, the diet was found to improve the patient's mental abilities compared to the effects of taking potassium bromide.

Also during the early 20th century, an American named Bernarr Macfadden popularized the idea of fasting as a means of restoring health. His student osteopath, Hugh Conklin, fasted introduced as a method of treatment to control epilepsy. Conklin proposed that epileptic seizures were caused by a secreted toxin in the gut and suggested that fasting for 18 to 25 days could cause the toxin to dissipate. His epilepsy patients were put on a "water diet," which reported healed 90% of children with the condition and 50% of adults. Analysis of the study that was performed later showed that, in fact, 20% of Conklin's patients became seizure-free, while 50% showed some improvement. Fasting therapy was soon adopted as part of mainstream therapy for epilepsy and in 1916, Dr.a New York medical journal that had successfully treated epileptic patients by prescribing a rapid, followed by a free starch and sugar diet since 1912.

It was in 1921 that the endocrinologist Rollin Woodyatt noticed that three water-soluble compounds, acetones, β-hydroxybutyrate and acetoacetate (called together ketone bodies) were produced by the liver as a result of starvation or followed a diet rich in fat and low in carbohydrates. Mayo Clinic's Wilder Russel called this "ketogenic diet" and used it as a treatment for epilepsy, also in 1921.

Further research in the 1960s showed that more ketones are produced by media-triglycerides (MCTs) by the energy unit because they are rapidly transported to the liver through the hepatic portal vein, as opposed to the lymphatic system. In 1971, Peter Huttenlocher devised a ketogenic diet where 60% of calories came from MCT oil, which allowed more protein and carbohydrates to be included compared to the original ketogenic diet, meaning that parents could prepare more enjoyable meals for their children with epilepsy. Many hospitals also adopted the MCT diet in lieu of the original ketogenic diet, although some used a combination of the two.

CHAPTER 01

WHAT IS KETOGENIC DIET

The ketogenic diet (or keto diet, in its abbreviated form) is a low-carbohydrate, high-fat diet that offers many health benefits.

In fact, about 20 studies show that this type of diet can help you lose weight and improve health.

Ketogenic diets can have benefits even against diabetes, cancer, epilepsy and Alzheimer's.

Below, we show a detailed guide for beginners about the keto diet.

What is a ketogenic diet?

The ketogenic diet is a low-carbohydrate, high-fat diet that shares many similarities with the Atkins and low-carb diets. This diet involves reducing carbohydrates drastically and replacing them with fats. This decrease exposes the body to a metabolic state called ketosis. When this happens, the body becomes incredibly efficient and manages to convert all the fat into energy. It also converts fat into ketones inside the liver, which can supply more energy to the brain. Ketogenic diets can cause reductions in blood sugar and insulin levels. This, together with the increase in ketones, provides numerous health benefits.

DIFFERENT TYPES OF KETOGENIC DIETS

With a popular diet, versions may tend to emerge. Currently, we are in nine types of the keto diet!

Wondering how many carbohydrates the foods you can eat and still be "in ketosis"? The traditional ketogenic diet created for those with epilepsy and is very strict with its percentages of macronutrients. But there are several other types of keto diet plans out there, as well. Let's see a second.

✓ The standard ketogenic diet (SKD): it consists of reaching approximately 75 per cent of calories from fat sources (such as oils or fattier cuts of meat), 5 per cent carbohydrates and 20% protein.

✓ The modified ketogenic diet (MKD): reducing carbohydrates, 30 per cent of your total caloric intake, while increasing fat and protein to 40 per cent and 30 per cent respectively

- ✓ The cyclic ketogenic diet (CKD): If you find it difficult to stick to a very low carbohydrate content of your daily diet, especially for months, you might want to consider a carb-cycling diet instead. Carb cycling increases the intake of carbohydrates (and sometimes the calories in general) only at the right time and in the right amounts, usually around 1 to 2 times per week (such as on weekends).

- ✓ The directed ketogenic diet (TKD): This plant eats simply tells you to follow the keto diet, BUT allows you to add carbohydrates around workouts. So on exercise days, you will be eating carbohydrates.

- ✓ The restricted ketogenic diet (RKD): Designed to treat cancer, this diet keto restricts calories as well as carbohydrates. Some studies indicate that caloric restriction and ketosis can help treat cancer.

- ✓ High protein ketogenic diet (HPKD): This version of the keto diet is often followed by people who want to preserve their muscle mass as bodybuilders and the elderly. Instead of protein making 20 per cent of the diet, here is 30 per cent. Meanwhile, fat goes up to 65 per cent of the diet and carbohydrates stay at 5 per cent. (Caution: people with kidney problems should not owe their protein too much.)

- ✓ The vegan ketogenic diet or a vegetarian diet: Yes, both are possible. Instead of products of animal origin, a lot of low carbohydrates, vegan nutrients and / or vegetarian foods are included. Nuts, seeds, low carb, fruits and vegetables, green leafy vegetables, healthy fats and fermented foods are all excellent choices in a plant-based diet keto. There is also a similar plan called ketotarian, which combines keto with vegetarian, vegan and / or pescatarian diets for supposedly greater health benefits.

✓ Dirty diet keto: «Dirty» is the apt term, as these of the version of keto follows the same strict percentages (75/20/5 of fat /protein/carbohydrates), but instead of focusing on healthy versions of fat, such as Coconut oil and wild salmon, you are free to eat naughtily, but still keto friendly with foods such as bacon, chorizo, pork rinds, diet sodas and so on. I DO NOT recommend this one.

✓ Lazy diet keto: Last but not least, the Lazy diet keto is often confused with the dirty keto ... but they are different, as the «lazy» refers to simply carefully tracking the fat and protein macros (or calories). Meanwhile, the only aspect that remains strict? Do not eat more than 20 grams of carbohydrates per day. Some people find this version less intimidating to start or end with ... but I warn you that your results will be less impressive.

How to Know Keto is Working (aka you are in Ketosis)

In the absence of glucose, which is normally used by cells as a quick source of energy, the body begins to burn fat and produces ketone bodies instead. Once the blood ketones levels rise to a certain point, you enter a state of ketosis, which generally results in rapid and steady weight loss until you reach a healthy, stable body weight. See this keto diet review, a before and after trying keto for 30 days.

To summarize a complex process, you get to this by burning fat when the liver breaks down fat into fatty acids and glycerol, through a process called beta-oxidation. There are three main types of ketone bodies, which are soluble in water, the molecules produced in the liver: acetoacetate, beta-hydroxybutyrate and acetone.

Thus, the body further breaks down these fatty acids into energy-rich in substances called ketones that circulate in the bloodstream. Fatty acid molecules that are metabolized through the process called ketogenesis, and a specific ketone body called acetoacetate is formed and that supplies energy.

The end result is to stay fueled out of high-level circulation of ketones (which are also sometimes called ketone bodies) - which is responsible for altering your metabolism in a way that some people, like to say it turns into a "fat burning machine." Both in terms of how you feel physically and mentally, along with the impact you have on the body, being in ketosis is very different from a " glycolytic state," where blood glucose (sugar) serves as the body of the energy source.

So, is ketosis bad for you? Of course not. If something is, it is the other way around. Many consider the burning of ketones to be much "cleaner" to maintain energy compared to the performance of carbohydrates and sugar on a day-to-day basis.

And remember, this state should not be confused with ketoacidosis, which is a serious complication of diabetes when the body produces an excess of ketones (blood or acids).

The goal is to keep in the east the fat burning in the metabolic state, in which you will lose weight until you reach your ideal set point. Some research suggests that this may be a new method to reverse diabetes naturally.

KETOGENIC DIETS CAN HELP YOU LOSE WEIGHT

A ketogenic diet is an effective way to lose weight and decrease risk factors in some diseases. In fact, research shows that the ketogenic diet outperforms the low-fat diets that are often recommended. Moreover, the goal of the diet is that you can lose weight without counting calories or track their intake. One study found that people who follow a ketogenic diet lose 2.2 times more weight than those who reduce calories and fat. Triglycerides and HDL cholesterol levels also show an improvement. Another study found that people with ketogenic diets lose 3 times more weight than those who follow traditional diets recommended. There are many reasons why the ketogenic diet is better than low-fat diets, such as the increase in protein intake, which provides numerous benefits. The increased ketones, the decrease in sugar levels and the improvement in insulin sensitivity could also play a key role.

KETOGENIC DIETS FOR DIABETES AND PREDIABETES

Diabetes is characterized by changes in metabolism, increase in blood sugar and deterioration in insulin functions. The ketogenic diet can help you lose excess fat, which is closely related to type 2 diabetes, prediabetes, and metabolic syndrome. One study found that the ketogenic diet improved insulin sensitivity by a huge 75% increase. In another study on people suffering from type 2 diabetes, it was found that 7 of the 21 participants were able to stop the use of all diabetes medications. In yet another study, the ketogenic group lost 24.4 pounds (11.1 kg), compared to the 15.2 pounds (6.9 kg) lost by the group with high carbohydrate intakes. It is an important benefit if we consider the relationship between weight and type 2 diabetes. Additionally, 95.2% of the ketogenic group was able to stop or reduce diabetes medicines, compared to 62% of the group with high carbohydrate intakes.

Other health benefits of the keto diet

The current ketogenic diet originated as a way to treat neurological diseases, such as epilepsy.

Some studies have shown that diet can have benefits in a wide variety of diseases:

- ✓ Cardiopathy: The ketogenic diet can improve risk factors such as body fat, HDL cholesterol levels, blood pressure and sugar present in the blood.

- ✓ Cancer: Currently, this diet has been used to treat many types of cancer and reduce the growth of tumors.

- ✓ Alzheimer's: Dietary keto could reduce Alzheimer's symptoms and slow down its progression.

- ✓ Epilepsy: Research has shown that the ketogenic diet can greatly reduce epileptic seizures in children.

- ✓ Parkinson: One study found that diet helped improve Parkinson's symptoms.

- ✓ Polycystic ovarian syndrome: The ketogenic diet can help reduce insulin levels, which could play a key role in polycystic ovarian syndrome.

- ✓ Brain injuries: A study in animals found that diet can reduce concussions and help the patient's recovery after suffering these injuries.

✓ Acne: The decrease in insulin levels and the reduction in the intake of sugar or processed foods could improve acne.

Foods to be avoided

Any food high in carbohydrates should be avoided.

✓ Here is a list of foods that should be reduced or eliminated in a ketogenic diet:

✓ Sugary foods: Soft drinks, fruit juices, smoothies, cakes, ice cream, sweets, etc.

✓ Cereals or starches: Products derived from wheat, rice, pasta, cereals, etc.

✓ Fruit: All fruits except small portions of berries, such as strawberries.

✓ Beans or legumes: Peas, red beans, lentils, chickpeas, etc.

✓ Vegetables root and tubers: Potatoes, sweet potatoes, carrots, parsnips, etc.

✓ Dietary or low-fat products: They are usually highly processed and rich in carbohydrates.

✓ Some condiments or sauces: Above all, those that contain sugar and saturated fats.

✓ Saturated fats: Limit the intake of refined oils, mayonnaise, etc.

✓ Alcohol: Due to its high carbohydrate content, many alcoholic beverages must be eliminated in a ketogenic diet.

✓ Dietary foods without sugars: They are usually rich in sugar alcohols, which can affect ketone levels. These foods also tend to be highly processed.

Foods to eat

You should base most of your meals around these foods:

✓ Meat: Red meat, ribeye, ham, sausage, bacon, chicken and turkey.

✓ Fatty fish: Like salmon, trout, tuna, and mackerel.

✓ Eggs: Look for eggs rich in omega 3 and pasteurized.

✓ Butter and cream: If possible, look for foods that have been fed grass.

✓ Cheese: Cheese not processed (cheddar, goat, creamy, blue or mozzarella).

✓ Nuts and seeds: Almonds, nuts, flax seeds, pumpkin seeds, chia seeds, etc.

✓ Healthy oils: Especially, extra virgin olive oil, coconut oil, and avocado oil.

✓ Avocado: Whole avocados or guacamole made naturally.

✓ Low carb vegetables: Most green vegetables, tomatoes, onions, and peppers, etc.

✓ Condiments: You can use salt, pepper, some herbs, and healthy spices.

It is better than the diet is based mainly on whole foods with a single ingredient.

What is the process of ketosis?

We must know that today carbohydrates are the main source of energy when they are ingested they go from the stomach to the intestine to disintegrate and become glucose that will be our fuel. Apart from the glucose present in our bloodstream, it is also stored in the form of glycogen in:

In the muscles: Deposit of approximately 200 grams of glycogen, this storage capacity depends a lot on the muscle mass that the specific person possesses and is used locally by each muscle demanding energy.

In the liver: Deposit of approximately 80 grams of glycogen, it is used as the second reserve after using the existing deposit in the musculature. It is also used as a general level for the correct functioning of the organism.

When all the glycogen reserves are depleted , our brain detects that there are no energy stocks to perform the required physical activity and it is then when the state of ketosis begins to occur, the so-called ketone bodies are released, these compounds cause the oxidation of the fats accumulated in our body to make use of them as a source of energy .

How long does it take to enter ketosis?

There is no specific time period to know when we are in ketosis, that is, to know when our body is burning accumulated fat to transform it into energy, the number of days necessary to enter ketosis is calculated between 3 and 7 days but it will depend on various factors; as the amount of glycogen that we have stored, the carbohydrate restriction that we carry out or the amount of exercise we perform. As explained,this diet is intended to reduce considerably the intake of carbohydrates and sugars, which are the main source of energy, since otherwise, it is not possible to enter the ketone state. We will spend only 10% of carbohydrates in the diet (when it is normally advised between 40% - 50% of the diet). They will consume around 50 grams of carbohydrates a day (which does not refer to the weight of the food, but to the number of carbohydrates that it has). We will not consume sugars, processed or refined foods. It is a diet with average protein intake, high in healthy fats and low in carbohydrates. Although the consumption of hydrates is low, we should never eliminate them completely. It is a diet that has some similarity with what our ancestors ate in the Paleolithic because at that time they ate meat and fish and did not eat too many carbohydrates such as pasta or cereals.

Why is it possible to lose weight with this Keto diet?

Normally we eat carbohydrates constantly in our diet and several times a day, the excess of carbohydrates and sugars in the diet causes the body to adapt to always using the glucose supplied as an energy source and the fats continue to be stored and not used.

With this diet what is intended is to put to work the fats that we have accumulated as the main source of energy thanks to the process of ketosis that we have just explained.

There are studies that show that fats are a slower energy source but more effective than carbohydrates. Each gram of carbohydrates becomes 4 kilocalories of energy, while each gram of fat becomes 9 kilocalories.

Advantages of diet

✓ Weight loss. Studies show that people who follow a diet low in carbohydrates lose more weight than those who follow a diet low in fat.

✓ Volume loss. In the first days the glycogen reserves are depleted (glycogen is formed by 1 molecule of glucose and 4 of water). If we have stored about 300 grams of glucose we will lose about 1,200 kilos of water. The loss of fat will come later.

✓ It does not produce hunger, it generates a high sensation of satiety due to the slower digestion of fats.

✓ It decreases the anxiety associated with other types of diets due to its high satiating power.

✓ Less amount of muscle loss compared to other diets due to its sufficient protein intake.

✓ It is Anti-inflammatory. Studies claim that the levels of pro-inflammatory cytokines are reduced when we enter ketosis

✓ It is anti-carcinogenic. The tumor cells need to metabolize large amounts of glucose to live, they can not survive with ketone bodies or fatty acids and they are toxic to them.

✓ More fat is lost from where we have more, usually from visible areas such as the abdomen, buttocks or thighs.

✓ Reduces blood sugar levels with great improvements for people suffering from type 2 diabetes.

✓ It helps to reduce the bad LDL cholesterol by the reduced intake of hydrates.

✓ It provides metabolic flexibility. Our body learns to use fats as an energy source, it becomes more efficient and later when hydrates are introduced they are managed more efficiently.

✓ The ketogenic diet mimics the effects that occur in our body biochemically when we do fasting, but without having to go hungry...

The phases of the ketogenic diet:

This diet for its functioning needs a metabolic change, and therefore we must adapt the organism to the new way of nourishing itself.

During the first week, we will change our diet significantly making it rich in fat, and poor in carbohydrates. During this week we can eat on demand. The weight loss during this week will not be significant, because at the beginning you will lose mostly fluids, but from the second week on you will begin to lose significant weight, as we will begin to lose accumulated fat.

During the second week we will eat on demand but with only two important meals a day, the rest will be small snacks. During this week, we will have to get used to not adding more fats to the food than our own. That is, we will not fry and consume foods cooked on the grill or steam. Not adding more fats than you already have. Once adopted the organism will feel with more energy.

CHAPTER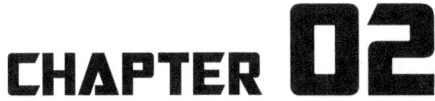

KETOGENIC FEEDING PLAN FOR 1 WEEK

To help you get started, here is an example of a food and ketogenic plan for 1 week:

Monday

Breakfast: Bacon, eggs, and tomatoes.

Lunch: Chicken salad with olive oil and feta cheese.

Dinner: Salmon with asparagus cooked in butter.

Tuesday

Breakfast: Eggs, tomatoes, basil, and goat cheese omelet.

Lunch: Almond milk, peanut butter, cocoa powder and milkshake with stevia.

Dinner: Meatballs, cheddar cheese, and vegetables.

Wednesday

Breakfast: A ketogenic milkshake.

Lunch: Seafood salad with olive oil and avocado.

Dinner: Pork chops with parmesan cheese, broccoli, and salad.

Thursday

Breakfast: Tortilla with avocado, sauce, peppers, onion, and spices.

Lunch: A handful of walnuts and celery sticks with guacamole and salsa.

Dinner: Chicken stuffed with pesto and cream cheese accompanied by vegetables.

Friday

Breakfast: Sugar-free yogurt with peanut butter, cocoa powder, and stevia.

Lunch: Veal sautéed and cooked in coconut oil with vegetables.

Dinner: Little burger made with bacon, egg, and cheese.

Saturday

Breakfast: Cheese and ham omelet with vegetables.

Lunch: Some slices of ham and cheese with walnuts.

Dinner: Whitefish, eggs, and spinach cooked in olive oil.

Sunday

Breakfast: Fried eggs with bacon and mushrooms.

Lunch: Hamburger with salsa, cheese, and guacamole.

Dinner: Fillets with eggs and salad.

Try to vary between vegetables and meat during the long season, as each one provides different nutrients and health benefits.

Ketogenic and healthy appetizers

In case you are hungry between meals, below you will find some ketogenic and healthy appetizers:

✓ Fatty meat or fish

- ✓ cheese

- ✓ A handful of nuts or seeds

- ✓ Cheese with olives

- ✓ 1 or 2 hard-boiled eggs

- ✓ Black chocolate 90%

- ✓ A low carb milkshake with almond milk, cocoa powder, and nut butter

- ✓ Whole milk yogurt with nut butter and cocoa powder

- ✓ Strawberries and cream

- ✓ Celery with salsa and guacamole

- ✓ Smaller portions of leftovers from meals

Tips for eating out and follow a ketogenic diet

It is not very difficult to find many restaurants with ketogenic foods when we go out to eat out. Most restaurants offer meat or fish dishes. You can order any of these foods and replace them with any meal rich in carbohydrates with extra vegetables. Meals with eggs are also a great option, as an omelet or eggs with bacon. Another ideal dish is a little burger. You could also replace the chips with vegetables. Add extra avocado, cheese, bacon or eggs. In some restaurants, you can enjoy any type of meat with extra cheese, guacamole, salsa, and sour cream. For dessert, you can order a table with assorted cheeses or fruits of the forest with cream.

Side effects and how to minimize them

Although the ketogenic diet is safe for healthy people, some side effects may appear at first until the body adapts. You can suffer the famous flu keto, which lasts a few days. The flu keto causes a decrease in energy and mental capacity, an increase in the sensation of hunger, sleep problems, nausea, digestive upset and decreased performance in exercise. To minimize this problem, you can try to follow a standard, low-carbohydrate diet during the first week. This could teach the body to burn more fat before it completely eliminates carbohydrates. A ketogenic diet can also change the balance of water and minerals in the body, so you can add extra salt to meals or take mineral supplements. In relation to minerals, try to take between 3,000 and 4,000 mg of sodium, 1,000 mg of potassium and 300 mg of magnesium per day to minimize side effects. At least at the beginning, it is important to eat until you feel full and avoid restricting too many calories. Normally, the ketogenic diet causes weight loss without intentional caloric reduction.

Supplements for a ketogenic diet

Although it is not necessary to take supplements, they can be useful.

- ✓ TMC oil: Add it to drinks or yogurt, as it provides energy and helps increase ketone levels.

- ✓ Minerals: Add salt and other minerals when the diet begins, as it may be important to balance water and mineral levels.

- ✓ Caffeine: Caffeine can have benefits for energy, fat loss, and performance.

- ✓ Exogenous ketones: This supplement may help increase the levels of ketone in the body.

- ✓ Creatine: Provides numerous benefits for health and performance. It can help if you combine a ketogenic diet with exercise.

- ✓ Whey protein: Pour half a tablespoon of whey protein in shakes or yogurt to increase daily protein intake.

Frequently asked questions

Here are some answers to the most frequently asked questions about the ketogenic diet.

1. Can I take carbohydrates again?

Yes, but it is important that you reduce carbohydrate intake significantly. After the first 2 or 3 months, you can eat hydrates on special occasions, but return to the diet immediately afterward.

2. Will I lose muscle?

There is a risk of losing muscle in any diet. However, high protein intake and ketone levels can help minimize muscle loss, especially if you lift weights.

3. Can I work the muscle on a ketogenic diet?

Yes, but it will not be as easy as on a moderate carb diet.

4. Do I need to do a carbohydrate refill?

No, but it may be beneficial to incorporate some days with more calories than normal.

5. How many proteins can I ingest?

Proteins should be moderate since high intake can cause spikes in insulin levels and decrease ketones. The maximum limit is probably the intake of 35% total calories.

6. What happens if I feel tired, weak or fatigued constantly?

It is possible that you are not performing the ketogenic diet properly or that your body does not use fats and ketones correctly. To counteract it, reduce carbohydrate intake and continue with the tips discussed above. It may also help to take TMC oil supplements or ketones.

7. Why does my urine smell like fruit?

Do not worry, it is simply due to the elimination of the products that are created during ketosis.

8. What can I do if my breath stinks?

It is a very common side effect. Try drinking water flavored with natural fruits or chew gum without sugar.

9. Is it true that ketosis is very dangerous?

People often confuse ketosis with ketoacidosis. The first is a natural procedure, while the second only occurs when there is uncontrolled diabetes.

Ketoacidosis is dangerous, but the ketosis that occurs during a ketogenic diet is perfectly normal and healthy.

10. What can I do if I have problems with digestion and diarrhea?

This side effect usually happens after 3 or 4 weeks. If it persists, try eating more fiber-rich vegetables. Magnesium supplements can also help with constipation.

REMEDIES FOR KETO DIET CONSTIPATION

If you have been following a ketogenic diet then you are already familiar with this eating plan with possible benefits, including losing weight, reducing blood pressure and better control of blood sugar. There are also some diet keto side effects to consider and once you know, you can easily make an effort to avoid them! One of these undesirable side effects is keto constipation diet. In general, constipation is a big problem for many people today. It is estimated that in the United States alone, chronic constipation results in 2.5 million doctor visits every year and the costs of medications reaching hundreds of millions of dollars.

Experiencing constipation is not pleasant, by any means and may include other unwanted symptoms from headaches to swelling of an irritable disposition. If you have been experiencing constipation in keto, it is time to fix this problem with truly effective natural remedies or avoid it in the first place.

Does the keto Diet Cause Constipation?

Constipation can be defined as the presence of difficulty in emptying the bowels and is usually associated with hardened stools. When you are constipated, the waste of food (stool) moves slower through the digestive tract.

The ketogenic diet is very low in carbohydrates, high in fat diet. Can a low carbohydrate diet cause constipation? It is possible, especially in the transition period when you change your previous eating habits for your new keto lifestyle. This is why it is so important to follow a keto diet in the healthiest way possible.

Many people are accustomed to getting their processed fibre "high in fibre" cereals before going to keto. After that switch to a keto diet and do not realize that there are still many healthy sources that are very low in carbohydrates, however, they have a lot of constipation-preventing fibre.

However, it is useful to know that keto constipation and diarrhoea can occur so much. It all depends on how your body reacts to your new diet. You can not experience any digestive symptom or you may experience diarrhoea instead of constipation. So does the keto diet do poop? For some people, this can increase bowel movements, but that is not always the case.

According to experts, at any time to make a big change in your diet, there is a possibility that they affect your gastrointestinal health. What's more, the whole colon world is unique, which is the reason why some people may be affected with constipation, others with diarrhoea, and even then, some may not notice a change at all. You are wondering, how can I avoid constipation in diet keto? I am about to tell you some of the best ways to prevent this side effect (which also includes keto constipation weight gain) so that you can really enjoy and experience the benefits of your new lifestyle keto!

How to get rid of constipation in keto? Cured keto constipation really is not difficult if you know the right food, beverages and supplements to include in your diet. Here are some of the best home remedies to start using today if you are following a keto diet and constipation has become a problem:

1. Hydration

Are you drinking enough water? It's so basic, but it's so important. If you are dehydrated, constipation is likely going to be a problem if you are following a keto diet or any other diet for that matter. Drink warm water or at room temperature, because this helps stimulate digestion better than very cold water. Drinking hot water with lemon on an empty stomach early in the morning can be particularly useful.

To increase your hydration level and encourage the step stool, you can also drink herbal teas, caffeinated teas including black and green, organic coffee in moderation and bone broth. It is especially important to increase your water intake when you are increasing your fibre intake because if you only add fibre and do not add more water to your diet, you can actually worsen constipation. You need moisturizing liquids to move the fibre along!

2. More Magnesium

If you are experiencing magnesium constipation keto it may be just what you need to get things moving again. Magnesium is essential for muscle relaxation. If you have a magnesium deficiency, then you are more likely to experience muscle tension, which may encourage constipation. Since ketosis can increase the washing of electrolytes, such as magnesium, from your system, it is very important that you avoid being deficient in magnesium. As a supplement, magnesium citrate (magnesium with citric acid) is the magnesium form best known for its laxative properties. You can also add more magnesium-rich foods that are diet-friendly keto on a daily basis.

3. Go Alkaline

Another way to combat any constipation, nausea or fatigue that develops in the transition to this new low carbohydrate lifestyle, you may want to consider adopting the keto-Alkaline diet. One of the key aspects of this version of the diet keto is that you, be sure to eat a lot of nutrients and rich in fibre, leafy green vegetables and good drinking water, which can not only help you to be more alkaline but can also help you avoid constipation

4. Sodium + Potassium

As just mentioned, electrolytes, such as potassium, sodium and magnesium can decrease faster when you enter ketosis. Not only can an electrolyte imbalance contribute to constipation as well as diarrhoea, but it can also cause headaches, cramps and general weakness. In addition to adding more magnesium to your keto diet, if you are experiencing constipation, you can also raise your potassium and sodium level.

A great keto-source of potassium is the delicious and very nutritious avocado. To ensure that your sodium levels are adequate, use a high-quality pink Himalayan sea salt to season the food. People often think of sodium or salt, like dehydration, but sodium in adequate amounts is the key to healthy water retention colon in a way that encourages optimal stool formation and elimination.

5. Wisely Chosen Fiber

They move on flakes, it's time to get your fibre of low carb, high density of nutrients from the elements that are keto-friendly like green leafy vegetables. To help prevent constipation keto, be sure to include high-fibre foods in your diet, especially vegetables. Although most of your calorie intake will be from vegetable fats they should be included in just about every meal you have while on the diet keto. The high fibre content of options that are keto-approved include:

✓ All vegetables without starch, especially green leafy vegetables, peppers, cruciferous vegetables such as broccoli or cauliflower, mushrooms, asparagus, zucchini, artichokes, etc.

✓ Avocado, which is a great source of fat, potassium and fibre.

✓ Coconut flakes/coconut flour, another high-fat source of fibre.

✓ Nuts (in small to moderate amounts) such as almonds, nuts, cashews, pistachios and Brazil nuts

✓ Seeds (in small to moderate quantities) that provide important nutrients include sesame, sunflower, chia, flax and pumpkin seeds.

6. Probiotics

If you are struggling with constipation probiotic keto should not be forgotten! You should include acceptable amounts of certain fermented foods in your diet on a regular basis. Rich in probiotics, fermented foods such as kefir, sauerkraut and kimchi are great keto-approved options that are loaded with beneficial probiotics that can help prevent and relieve constipation.

7. Exercise

There is a large number of diet adjustments that you can make to your keto diet to discourage the onset of constipation, but do not forget the most important thing that you can do physically to avoid this unpleasant symptom - exercise! The lack of physical activity can undoubtedly contribute to constipation.

By exercising regularly, you are not only accelerating the movement of your body; You are also speeding the movement of your bowels. Aerobic exercise, in particular, encourages the natural by tightening the muscles of the intestine, which is necessary for the passage of stool.

Final thoughts

Making a major change in your diet can result in temporary digestive problems such as constipation.

✓ If you decide to go to keto and constipation becomes a problem, there are many easy adjustments you can make to your diet to get rid of this unwanted side effect.

✓ Not everyone experiences constipation while following a keto diet; Some people have diarrhoea, while others do not deal with any of the symptoms.

✓ You can improve and prevent keto swelling and constipation:

✓ Stay hydrated with plenty of hot / water at room temperature. You can also drink herbal teas, caffeinated teas including black and green, organic coffee in moderation and bone broth.

✓ Make sure you have enough electrolytes (magnesium, potassium and sodium) in your diet.

✓ Opt for an alkalized version of the ketogenic diet and consume a lot of keto-friendly fibre like green leafy vegetables.

✓ Eat foods rich in probiotics, such as kefir and kimchi and also take a probiotic supplement.

✓ Exercise regularly, especially aerobic exercise.

PRECAUTIONS WHEN A KETOGENIC DIET IS FOLLOWED

Remember, the ketogenic diet will really change your metabolism, which put you into ketosis, and turn from a sugar burner to a fat burner. Those are significant changes in your body, and you are bound to notice some symptoms of the so-called flu keto.

Keto flu symptoms may include tiredness, difficulty sleeping, digestive problems such as constipation, weakness during workouts, being in a bad mood, losing libido and bad breath. Fortunately, these side effects do not affect everyone and often last only 1 to 2 weeks. In general, the symptoms disappear when the body gets used to being in ketosis. If a ketogenic diet is being used by a child to treat epilepsy, strict medical supervision is necessary. If you are very active and without much fat in your body, consider trying carbohydrate cycling or at least eating a modification of the keto diet that does not severely restrict carbohydrate intake.

Ketogenic diets were originally developed to help improve the symptoms of epilepsy (specifically in children who do not improve with other treatments), but today very low carbohydrate diets are used to help adults, including those who suffer from many other chronic health problems such as obesity, cancer and diabetes. Fast and reliable weight loss for people who follow a ketogenic diet is due to a decrease in insulin levels and the body is forced to burn stored body fat for energy

CHAPTER 03

INTERMITTENT FASTING

Fasting has been practiced since time immemorial. In origin for religious or health reasons, (even animals practice it) in recent years has been practiced in different versions to lose weight or as a detox diet. The latest dietary fashion goes through fasting much more moderate and bearable than that of yesteryear. Your practice can greatly benefit the body.

What is intermittent fasting

Intermittent fasting consists of leaving the body deprived of food for some hours of the day, extending the time that goes from dinner to breakfast. This interval, according to his followers, should be at least twelve hours each day: that is, if you usually eat dinner at nine o'clock at night, you should not eat breakfast or eat any kind of food until nine o'clock in the morning. Little by little this time should be lengthening, to be able to arrive at fourteen or sixteen hours without food, at least during some days of the week.

BENEFITS OF INTERMITTENT FASTING FOR HEALTH

There are benefits of fasting that will help keep your body healthy and receive positive effects on your mental and physical health. Although yes, and which is very important: before doing so it is recommended that you consult a doctor and do a review.

In a world where the body is an important factor when developing and relating, the desire to constantly improve our physique sometimes becomes something sick and obsessive

One of the main complexes is to spend the kilos that a priori "is appropriate" for society and that is why they are constantly reinventing new formulas to be able to leave behind the unwanted weight.

The benefits offered by fasting are several, among which is developed especially in the moments referred to ketosis (body situation in which our body is induced to a state based on low carbohydrate index).

Commonly known as "miraculous cure", below we will explain the benefits of carrying out this action, and as always, with caution and head.

1- Help to lose weight

The first and most clear of all is the help that gives us to lose weight. Whenever it is controlled within a certain time throughout the day, fasting will help our body to be able to burn fat in a much faster and of course, effective way.

2- Prevention of type 2 diabetes

According to a study published in 2005 by the Journal of Applied Physiology, after fasting periods, insulin acts more effectively when it comes into contact with blood cells. Therefore fasting improves the sensitivity of our body against insulin.

All this has as a consequence the protection against the appearance of diabetes, specifically, type 2 diabetes.

According to a study published in 2014 by Medical News Today, the 1-day fasting, only taking water, can reduce in high probabilities the risk of suffering from type 2 diabetes.

3- Accelerates the metabolism

Fasting makes burning fat much more quickly and effectively, which is because our metabolism is accelerated by the lack of food to convert, and also helps maintain a much less forced intestinal function and therefore, more healthy.

4- Increase in life expectancy

Diet has a lot of influence over the years and the life expectancy of people. It is scientifically proven that people who reduce their diet in greater quantities live longer than those who eat more than enough food.

It is said that the Indian or Peruvian cultures are the longest due to the diet that they continue within their borders.

5- Prevents cancer

It should be noted that this benefit is not proven one hundred percent, but it is true that there is promising evidence in practices with animals and several humans.

The results have concluded that fasting is an extra help to chemotherapy as well as alleviating its side effects.

6- Improve the immune system

According to a study conducted by experts, fasting creates a kind of "reboot" by which our immune cells are purified and cleaned up and regenerates the oldest ones. In this way, protection against cell damage is produced, which leads to the following benefit.

7- Improves and protects the skin

Being long periods of time without our body having to divert an important focus of energy to digestion we can redirect it towards the regeneration of other organic systems.

One of the organs that improve is skin. Our toxins are cleaned, avoiding among many other effects, the appearance of acne or different black spots. In addition, it also improves the functioning of organs such as the liver or kidneys among others.

8- Improves the state of the heart

A fast for several hours will lead to a direct reduction of several risk factors related to the heart since there will be direct changes in our blood pressure or cholesterol.

Some dangers to consider

It is necessary to take into account a series of negative consequences that may arise at the time of carrying out this process.

- ✓ Dehydration: Produced due to lack of food consumption.

- ✓ Headache: Derived from dehydration. The headaches can get accentuated with the passage of time.

✓ Weakness: Physically we will be exhausted, so it is convenient not to do much physical exercise.

✓ Heartburn: During this period, our stomach will produce higher than normal amounts of acid.

THE METHOD OF INTERMITTENT FASTING TO LOSE WEIGHT QUICKLY

Although the word ' fasting ' may seem very drastic, it is true that maintaining a specific meal schedule influences fat burning or accumulation. This does not mean that we have to go hungry, intermittent fasting refers to building a food pattern in which we eat at certain times only.

Ingesting calories during a specific period of the day, stopping eating a certain number of hours, is shown to help you lose weight, but you have to know how to do it.

Normally, our body uses glucose or glycogen for energy. When we do not consume food for several hours (at least 12-16), in our body begins a process called ketogenesis, which uses stored fat to give energy to the body. That is, during a prolonged fasting period, the accumulated fat is burned and not muscle, as it happens in some other weight loss diets.

What is the method of intermittent fasting? Well, simply choose a time section in the day to not consume food and make the intake in the hours that are outside of that stretch. The most widespread is a period of 16 hours of fasting with 8 hours of food intake, although there are also people who perform intermittent fasting for 24 hours from time to time to maintain their weight and to give a rest to their body and increase their Energy. In the case of women, you could also do an intermittent fast 12/12, that is, you can dine at 9 pm and have breakfast the next day at 9 am in the morning. You would be 12 hours without eating and another 12 eating.

In any case, calorie restriction is very important to lose weight and intermittent fasting is usually an implicit consequence of reducing the number of hours we eat. This point, added to that promotes insulin sensitivity and increases the secretion of growth hormone, are key to lose weight.

The intermittent fasting 16: 8 works but you also have to be aware that in the hours in which it is allowed to eat the ideal is to opt for healthy and quality food. Do not take advantage to put in your window of food very processed or very caloric, since in such a case you would not notice the benefits of burning fat from fasting. If in the hours that you can eat you end up pulling pizza, burgers or fried, you will not lose weight. If, on the other hand, you maintain a healthy and balanced diet based on vegetables, good fats and proteins, you will find in the intermittent fasting a great ally to lose weight. This eating pattern also improves the immune system and protects against cancer and neuronal degeneration. Even some studies suggest that it could increase longevity. Do you need more reasons to prove it?

This practice is very old and very safe, it is not a miracle diet, nor is it a fad, we are designed for it. In Ancient Greece, their virtues were already practiced and applauded. It helps to restore balance in our body, helping you to burn fat during periods of fasting. With intermittent fasting in addition to losing weight, you will simplify your life and gain health.

ADVANTAGES OF INTERMITTENT FASTING

Besides benefits for body composition or weight loss, there are a number of advantages that accompany intermittent fasting.

Easier to manage than traditional dieting: Preparing a single (or a couple, depending on your feeding window) meals per day is logistically easier than preparing several meals from a time management standpoint. Plus, intermittent fasting saves you the headache of rigorous meal prepping or finding foods that comply with a specific diet.

The decrease in fat mass: Individuals who practiced intermittent fasting showed a decrease in fat mass while maintaining muscle mass and strength.

Longevity: Studies have shown that populations who fast on a regular basis can appear to have increased longevity. A study was performed on rats that ate only once per day and it found that compared to other groups, those rats had a longer lifespan regardless of the amount of food consumed.

Improved health and metabolism: Metabolic health may be improved with fasting by way of circadian biology, gut microbiome, and modifiable lifestyle behaviors, such as sleep. Research has shown that intermittent fasting may help improve blood lipids, glycemic control, control insulin levels, decrease blood pressure, and decrease inflammation.

Boost brain health: Fasting robustly is a strong trigger for neurogenesis and beta-hydroxybutyrate (or BHB, one of the three ketone bodies), which can trigger the release of brain growth factors.

Speed up endurance adaptation: Fasting promotes pathways involved in fat metabolism, which may help endurance performance—for example, growth of new mitochondria.

Reduced risk of diabetes: Through intermittent fasting, reduced insulin resistance can help those with type 2 diabetes lower blood glucose levels and improve blood sugar. Intermittent fasting can also decrease inflammation

SCIENCE BEHIND INTERMITTENT FASTING

When you consume carbohydrates, the pancreas begins to release insulin-triggering carb uptake and storage.

Carbohydrates in our food (and to a lesser extent, protein) trigger the release of the hormone. The insulin, in turn, tells the body to store any excess energy as glycogen or as fat for later use. Some of the fat is stored in the liver, but most of it becomes fat deposits in the body. Insulin also switches off the processes that release fat from fat deposits, meaning that fat is going into storage and not used as fuel.

When you practice intermittent fasting, on the other hand, energy intake is lower, insulin levels begin to fall and fat burning increases.

By increasing the amount of time the body is in a fasted state, there will be more time for the body to tap into stored energy. Across evolution, most species would regularly enter a fasted state. Predators tend to eat larger portions at one given time and may not consume food for several days. There is nothing wrong with occasionally fasting for longer periods of time and it actually has several health benefits (but of course, consult your doctor before doing this).

Caloric Restriction

Simply put, restricting the number of calories you consume will put the body into a fasted state.

There is a common belief that skipping a meal is bad for your metabolism or overall health. Truth is, we're seeing more data support the idea of restricted eating. The three-meals-a-day convention has been standard in American diets for decades. But obesity has increased. Diabetes and pre-diabetes have also increased.

In studies performed on animals,those in a fasted state had longer lifespans compared to those that did not fast. It seems the benefits of fasting can not only be seen short term but over the course of a lifetime as well.

An interesting diet that mimics fasting is called the Prolon Diet. The idea is to really decrease insulin release while still providing nutrients. It's a low-protein, low-carbohydrate, high-fat diet with calorie intake ranging from 770 - 1,100 calories per day. Studies have shown a fast-mimicking diet can improve biomarkers for aging, diabetes and cardiovascular disease.

CHAPTER 04

MAINTAINING A LOW CARB HIGH-FAT DIET

HISTORY IN BRIEF

Researchers show that the low-carbohydrate, high-fat diet promotes faster weight loss than the low-fat diet. People who ate low-carbohydrate diet lost 10 pounds in 45 days, while those who ate low-fat diet needed 70 days to lose the same amount of weight

The keys to a successful weight loss and prevention of diseases related to diabetes and heart disease are severe restrictions of refined carbohydrates from sugar to grains, along with higher levels of saturated fats.

The conventional advice has focused on low-fat diets for weight loss and prevention of heart disease, but again and again, researchers are now confirming that refined carbohydrates of sugars and grains are the main culprits behind the high rates of obesity, along with related diseases , such as diabetes, heart disease and cancer.

The historical data also clearly show that when they traditionally abandoned their traditional food for a Western-style diet, they inevitably began to suffer from these health problems, even though they had been practically non-existent in their culture.
You simply have to address the issue of carbohydrates in your diet in order to successfully control your weight and improve your health ...

In a recent study,reseachers confirmed this theory, when they compared the effects of two diets on vascular health; one low in fat, the other low in carbohydrates.

A total of 46 men and women weighing an average of 218 pounds participated in the study. The six-month-long weight loss program consisted of moderate aerobic exercise and strength training and one of two diets, either:

- ✓ Low-carbohydrate, high-fat diet: Less than 30 per cent of the calories from carbohydrates (pasta, bread and sugary fruits) and up to 40 per cent of fat (meat, dairy products and nuts)

- ✓ low-fat diet, high-carbohydrate diet: Less than 30 per cent of calories from fat and 55 per cent of carbohydrates.

The low-carb group on average lost 10 pounds in 45 days, while the low-fat group took 70 days to lose the same amount of weight. Regarding vascular health, the low-carbohydrate but high-fat group did not show harmful vascular changes, which is the main reason why many people are afraid of high-fat diets.

Two Keys to Stop Uncontrolled Obesity

If you want to lose excess weight or maintain an ideal weight, you need:

- ✓ Restrict severely carbohydrates (sugars, fructose and grains), and

- ✓ Increase the consumption of healthy fats

One of the easiest ways to achieve this is to move your diet away from processed foods and include one based on whole foods (preferably organic). This way, you will automatically avoid the GREAT amounts of fructose, which is one of the four main sources of calories.

If you develop the habit of reading labels, you will find that high fructose corn syrup (HFCS) is in almost everything - including foods you would never expect, such as diet foods, "improved" water products, and even baby formulas.

It would also be wise to radically reduce the number of refined grains in your diet, such as breakfast cereals, bread, rolls, cookies and more, as these are rapidly broken down into sugar, which would raise insulin levels and cause resistance to insulin.

It is important to remember that insulin resistance is the main underlying factor of almost all chronic diseases known to man, including heart disease. Avoiding all kinds of cereal-based products will also automatically help avoid trans fat that damage health, which is found in high amounts in baking products.

As you reduce or eliminate refined carbohydrates from your diet, be sure to increase your fat intake and yes, that means saturated fat. (Again, avoid trans fats, such as margarine and vegetable oils, as they are the ones that cause cardiovascular health problems most commonly associated with saturated fats.)

Saturated fats are not only good for you; They are essential for proper cellular and hormonal function. They also provide a concentrated source of energy in your diet - a source of energy that is more ideal than carbohydrates - which is why I chose these two specific "keys" in combination because when you reduce carbohydrates, you usually need to increase your fat intake. However, while food grains and sugars increase insulin levels and promote insulin resistance, eating fats do not.

Keep in mind that you should not eliminate vegetable carbohydrates from your diet. When talking about harmful carbohydrates, we are only referring to grains and sugars. On the contrary, you need to radically increase the number of vegetables you eat, because, in volume, the grains you replace are denser than the vegetables. To guide you on the right path, review my Nutrition Plan, which takes you slowly through these dietary changes.

How Fructose Causes Obesity and Poor Health

I want to put special emphasis on fructose as a source of carbohydrates that should be strictly controlled because fructose is the worst of all. Thanks to the excellent work of researchers, we now know that fructose:

- ✓ It is metabolized differently to glucose and most of it is converted directly into fat

- ✓ Tricks your body by making it gain weight by turning off the system that controls the appetite. Fructose does not adequately stimulate insulin, which in turn does not suppress ghrelin (the "hunger hormone") and does not stimulate leptin (the "satiety hormone"), which together make it eat more and develop resistance to insulin

- ✓ It leads quickly to weight gain and abdominal obesity ("beer belly"), lowers HDL, increases LDL, raises triglycerides, raises blood sugar levels and high blood pressure, that is, the classic metabolic syndrome.

- ✓ Over time it causes insulin resistance, which is not only an underlying factor of type 2 diabetes and heart disease but also many types of cancer.

Carbohydrates make us fat, right? This common mistake comes from the claim that carbohydrates are bad for us because they are converted to glucose, causing the release of insulin, which helps the body store any excess energy in the form of fat. However, it is not only carbohydrates that stimulate the secretion of insulin, proteins and high-fat food, they also do so. In fact, but too much energy from any nutritious source will also lead to weight gain.

Over the years there have been many versions of the low-carbohydrate, high-fat diet (the LCHF diet), eg Atkins, Dukan and the most recent, the ketogenic diet, but all have the same diet model: a very low carbohydrate intake (approximately 20-50 g per day), high in fat and moderate protein intake. Diets usually involve the exclusion of grains, legumes, dairy products, refined sugar and most starchy fruits and vegetables. The carbohydrates in these diets come from non-starchy vegetables, nuts and seeds. The LCHF diet defends the claim that diets can help you lose weight, control hunger and improve health. Some confirm that LCHF diets can be used as a cancer treatment.

Is there any science that supports these claims?

Research shows that, when carefully planned, the LCHF diet can be an effective treatment for people suffering from epilepsy and can help control type 2 diabetes. There is also evidence that very low carbohydrate diets can result in greater weight loss for obese people compared to low-fat diets. However, any weight loss that occurs is probably the result of the lack of calories created by the exclusion of energy-rich food and follow an extremely low-carbohydrate diet could be for many people a not so practical and long-term sustainable option term. In addition, many carbohydrates found in food, such as fruits, vegetables and whole grains, contain important components for health, including vitamins, minerals and dietary fibre.

Although the use of the ketogenic diet (the LCHF diet) in the treatment of cancer has shown promising results, it is necessary to do a deeper investigation to better explain the effects. The limited number of studies and the differences in their designs and characteristics, which end up giving evidence of low quality, make it very difficult to draw a firm conclusion, based on the facts.

How do carbohydrates fit into a healthy diet?

The carbohydrates are a type of macronutrients found in most foods and are a very important part of our diets. They are converted into glucose, which the body uses as a source of energy to maintain the functioning of muscles and organs. Various types of carbohydrates are differentiated by chemical composition, speed of digestion and absorption:

✓ Simple carbohydrates are made up of one or two sugar molecules and are rapidly digested and absorbed by our body. The added sugar and sugar found in fruits or milk are examples of simple carbohydrates.

✓ Complex / starchy carbohydrates are made up of a long chain of sugar and take longer to digest. Examples of complex carbohydrates include potatoes, legumes and whole grains eg brown rice, barley and oats.

✓ Dietary fibre is carbohydrate of plant origin that differs from simple or complex carbohydrates because it is not digested in the small intestine and, therefore, reaches the large intestine. Fibre helps keep our digestive system healthy and prevent constipation.

Foods rich in fibre, such as fruits or vegetables, wholemeal bread/pasta, nuts and seeds can help maintain weight because they can give the feeling of fullness and satiety.

The European Food Safety Authority (EFSA for its acronym in English) recommends a carbohydrate intake of between 45 and 60 per cent within the total energy intake, both for adults and children and the World Health Organization (WHO) recommends that less than 10% of carbohydrate consumption should come from free sugars. Eating a variety of foods that contain carbohydrates gives the maximum nutritional benefit.

Research shows that eliminating unnecessarily a group of foods from the diet can lead to a deficiency of nutrients and create a negative relationship with food, which can cause, in extreme cases, an eating disorder. It is important to remember that the balance, variety and control of the rations is the key.

BENEFITS AND RISKS OF A LOW CARBOHYDRATE DIET

It became famous for the Atkins Diet and other similar weight-loss plans for low-carb diets are best known for shedding pounds fast. And despite what might initially come to mind when thinking about low carb diet plans - for example, eating loads of meat, cheese, oil and butter - research suggests that a balanced low diet Carbohydrates pose some health risks if done well.

In fact, certain low-carbohydrate diets, such as the ketogenic diet, have been shown not only to be very effective for weight loss but also to improve the health of markers such as blood sugar levels as well as neurological health, hormonal balance and more. A low carb diet is a diet that limits carbohydrates in foods, such as foods with added sugar, grains, starchy vegetables and fruits - and emphasizes foods high in protein and fat.

Low-carbohydrate diets are nothing new and have been used in the medical community for a variety of purposes for more than a century. Based on decades of research, low-carbohydrate diets have been linked to the benefits, including:

✓ rapid weight loss

✓ the reduction of hunger

✓ better control over insulin and blood sugar

✓ improved cognitive performance

✓ lower risk of heart disease factors

✓ Reducing the risk of certain types of cancer

The benefits of low carb diets are mainly due to a reduction, or in some cases almost a complete elimination of glucose. Glucose or other molecules that can turn into glucose once eaten are found in all carbohydrate-rich foods - whether cereals, legumes, starchy vegetables, fruits and sweeteners of all kinds. To a lesser degree, even nuts, seeds and vegetables contain glucose.

How to make low-carbohydrate diets? They are effective because they cause glucose to run quickly, and when your supply is low enough, your body converts fat as fuel as a backup source - whether it is fats from your diet, or your own body fat stored.

Our bodies normally run on glucose or sugar for energy, but we can not make glucose on ourselves and only store about 24 hours in our muscles and in the liver. Once the carbohydrate glucose is not available for your energy because of the following low-carb diet, we start to burn the stored fat to get fuel instead. This is why low carb diets often lead to rapid weight loss and other metabolic improvements within a relatively short period of time.

THE DIFFERENCE BETWEEN LOW DIETS IN CARBOHYDRATES: HIGH-FAT CONTENT VS. HIGH PROTEIN

People can mean different things when it comes to low carbohydrate diets, which creates some confusion about what a low carb diet might actually look like. For example, what type of low carb diet is most common and most beneficial, high in fat or high protein?

High in Fats, Low in Carbohydrates Diets (also known as the Ketogenic Diet):

A ketogenic diet - a form of the very low carbohydrate content of the diet is a high-fat diet that strictly eliminates almost all sources of glucose in order to put the body in "fat-burning mode," also called nutritional of ketosis. The ketogenic diet goes by several different names, including the "non-carb diet" or "very low carbohydrate ketogenic diet" (LCKD or VLCKD for short).

Ketogenic diets have been used by doctors to treat patients with epilepsy and metabolic diseases since the 1920s! Benefits have been documented, such as helping treat epilepsy, promoting rapid weight loss and reducing the risk of diabetes. Not only do they have studies during the last century shows that the keto diet can reduce the amount of attacks patients suffer, but it can also have positive effects on the body fat, blood sugar, cholesterol levels, levels of Hunger and neurological health.

✓ When you are following a traditional ketogenic diet, you consume about 75 per cent of your daily calories from healthy fats, only about 5 per cent carbohydrates, and about 20 per cent protein.

✓ The ketogenic diets limit net daily carbohydrate consumption to only 20-30 grams (net carbohydrates are the number of carbohydrates left over when the fibre is subtracted from total carbohydrates).

✓ While the keto diet is a great fit for the type of person, many people still experience great results when eating a modification of the keto diet that is slightly higher in carbohydrates, or "keto-cycling" or " carb " -cycling »in which to boost the consumption of carbohydrates on certain days of the week.

✓ Compared to high protein diets, the ketogenic diet is considered "moderate protein." It is important not to over-consume protein in the keto diet as this may interfere with its ability to produce ketone bodies for energy and to enter in nutritional ketosis.

You might be concerned about how restrictive a ketogenic diet is going to be, and maybe you are worried about the side effects or "carb removal". Initially, keto diets can cause some side effects that usually last from 1 to 2 weeks.

However, data from certain clinical trials have shown that low-carbohydrate diets, even very low-carbohydrate ketogenic diets, can actually help improve mood and reduce fatigue and hunger. A 2007 study conducted by the Department of Psychiatry and Behavioral Sciences at Duke University Medical Center found that participants experienced significant improvements in a wide range of negative symptoms when following a very low carbohydrate content of the diet, even more than participants after a low-fat diet. Those in the very low carbohydrate content reported less fatigue, cognitive symptoms, the physical effects of hunger, insomnia and stomach problems than the low-fat diet group.

High Protein, Low Carbohydrate Diets:

Generally speaking, people who are not intentionally controlling their proteins usually take about 15-25 per cent of their daily calories from protein foods.

If you choose to follow a high protein diet, your diet will be more or less distributed from 30 to 35 per cent protein, 20% or less of carbohydrates, and around 45 to 50 per cent fat. With each meal, you'll want to incorporate 1-2 palm-sized portions of protein, such as fish or meat.

The main difference between high-fat content and high protein diets is the amount of protein in the form of meat, fish, eggs, etc. - that someone is eating. More fat diets such as the keto diet calls for more healthy fats in the form of butter, oil and fattier cuts of meat, while those on higher protein diets include fats, but less.

What Can You Eat on a Low-Carbohydrate Diet?

Amount of carbohydrates you should eat in a day on a low carb diet?

Depending on who you ask, a low carb diet can include any diet that consists of less than 30 to 40 per cent of the daily calories/energy of the carbohydrates.

Forty per cent of your diet consisting of carbohydrates is still a relatively high amount, so if you dedicate yourself to eating low carb, you probably want to consume much less than this. On the other hand, low-fat diets are those that involve obtaining 25 to 30 per cent or less of the daily calories/energy of the fat.

✓ Each person is different, but in general, the reduction of carbohydrates of about 30 per cent of their total diet, while the increase of fat to 40 per cent protein and 30 per cent, is a great goal to what to aim

✓ From there, you can choose to further adjust your macronutrients intake ("macronutrients" are fats, carbohydrates and proteins) to reach certain goals, for example, enter ketosis through a ketogenic diet.

✓ So, how many carbohydrates are included in a low carb diet? If you eat 2,000 to 2,500 calories per day, getting 30 per cent of your daily calories from carbohydrates equals about 150 grams to 187 grams of carbohydrates per day (each gram of carbohydrates contains approximately 4 calories).

✓ This amount can be considered to be relatively low in carbohydrates, although carbohydrates are still much higher then you want to eat on a diet like the ketogenic diet.

The best way to start eating a lower carbohydrate content of the diet is to simply focus on eliminating the main sources of added sugar and carbohydrates - especially from sugar snacks, sugary drinks, cereals and, possibly, legumes and dairy products, too. At the same time, work on increasing calories from healthy fats and quality proteins. Following these guidelines, most adults will see rapid weight loss and improvements in overall health.

Keep in mind that each person reacts differently to different dietary plans, and there is not necessarily a one-size-fits-all approach to the low carb diet that will work best for everyone. Factors such as that of someone of your age, gender, activity level, body weight and genetic predisposition affect the way that person feels when following a low carb diet.

Therefore, it is important to practice self-awareness if you are going to reduce your carbohydrate intake in order to get to the level of carbohydrates in your diet that works best for you personally. This may take a bit of trial and error initially, and it is best to reduce the carbohydrates gradually to avoid side effects such as the urge to be tired.

What can you eat on a low carb diet?

1. Healthy Fats

Most healthy fats contain zero net carbohydrates, especially the types listed below, which also has other health benefits.

Fats should be included in high quantities at every meal throughout the day.

✓ Healthy fats include saturated fats, monounsaturated fats and certain types of polyunsaturated acids (Agri), especially omega-3 fatty acids. It is best to include all types in your diet, with an emphasis on saturated fats, especially when compared to Agri.

✓ MCT oil, cold pressed coconut, palm fruit, olive oil, flaxseed, macadamia nuts and avocado oil, butter and ghee, avocado, lard, chicken fat or duck fat, all are good options

2. Quality Proteins

The proteins of animal origin (meat, fish, etc.) have very little, if any, carbohydrates. You can consume in moderate amounts as necessary to control hunger. In general, choose organic, grass-fed and fattier cuts of meat instead of the thinnest ones. For example, chicken thighs and legs are preferable to chicken breasts, since they contain much more fat.

✓ The grass-fed beef and other types of fatty cuts of meat, lamb, goat, beef, venison and other game. Fed with grass, fatty meat is preferable because it is higher in the quality of omega-3 fats.

✓ Organ meats, including the liver

✓ Poultry, including turkey, chicken, quail, pheasant, hen, goose, duck

✓ Free cage of eggs and egg yolks

✓ Fish, such as tuna, trout, anchovies, sea bass, sole, mackerel, salmon, sardines, etc.

3. The Vegetables Without Starch

✓ All green leafy vegetables, including dandelion or beet greens, kale, mustard greens, turnip, arugula, chicory, endive, escarole, fennel, chicory, romaine lettuce, sorrel, spinach, kale, chard, etc.

✓ Cruciferous vegetables such as broccoli, cabbage, Brussels sprouts and cauliflower

✓ Celery, cucumber, zucchini, spring onion and leek

✓ Fresh herbs

✓ Vegetables that are slightly higher in carbohydrates (but still low considering all things) include asparagus, mushrooms, bamboo shoots, bean sprouts, pepper, peas, water chestnuts, radishes, jicama, green beans, wax of beans, tomatoes

✓ The avocado (technically a fruit)

4. Dairy Rich in Fat

Dairy products should be limited to just «now and then» because they contain natural sugars. High in fat, hard cheeses have fewer carbohydrates, while low-fat milk and soft cheeses have much more.

✓ Of cow fat and goat milk (ideally organic and raw materials) and fat of the cheese.

5. Appetizers

✓ Bone broth (homemade or protein powder)

✓ Beef or turkey jerky

✓ Boiled eggs

✓ Extra vegetables (raw or cooked) with homemade dressing

✓ 1/2 avocado with slices of smoked salmon (salmon)

✓ Minced meat wrapped in lettuce

6. Condiments

✓ Spices and herbs, hot sauce, apple cider vinegar, sugar-free mustards, cocoa, powder, vanilla extract, stevia

7. Drinks

✓ Water, sugar-free coffee (black) and fresh tea made from vegetable juice and bone broth

Food to eat in limited quantities

You will want to limit foods such as starchy vegetables that contain more carbohydrates (such as peas, artichokes, okra, carrots, beets and turnips, sweet potatoes and potatoes), legumes, grains, fruits and dairy products such as yoghurt/kefir.

The amount you have of these will depend on how low carbohydrate content of the diet you are following. As a general rule, no more than 1/2 cup of cooked grains per day.

What Not to Eat in a Low-Carbohydrate Diet?

1. Any type of sugar

✓ White, coffee, cane, raw and impalpable sugar

✓ Syrups such as maple, carob, corn, caramel and fruit

✓ And of agave honey

✓ Any food made with ingredients such as fructose, glucose, maltose, dextrose and lactose

2. Any and All Grains

A slice of bread or a small portion of grains can have between 10-30 net grams of carbohydrates! Cereals and cooked grains usually have 15 to 35 grams per 1/4 cup of crude, depending on the species.

✓ Wheat, oats, all rice (white, brown, jasmine), quinoa, couscous, rice, etc.

✓ Corn and all products that contain corn, including popcorn, corn tortillas, corn grits, polenta and corn flour

✓ All kinds of products made with flour, including bread, bagels, bread, pasta, etc.

3. Almost All Processed Foods

✓ Cookies, french fries, pretzels, etc.

✓ All types of sweets

✓ All desserts such as cookies, cakes, pies, ice cream

✓ Pancakes, waffles and other breakfast items

✓ Oatmeal and cereals

✓ Snack on carbohydrates, granola bars, most protein bars or meal replacements, etc.

✓ Canned soups, packaged foods, any pre-packaged food

✓ Foods that contain artificial as well as artificial ingredients, sweeteners (sucralose, aspartame, etc.), colours and flavours

4. Sweets and Caloric Drinks

✓ Soda

✓ Alcohol (beer, wine, liquor, etc.)

✓ Sweetened teas or coffee drinks

✓ Milk and milk substitutes (cow's milk, soy milk, almond milk, coconut milk, Lactaid, cream, half and half, etc.)

✓ The fruit juices.

Can you eat the fruit on a low carb diet? If so, which fruit has fewer carbohydrates? Berries, including blueberries, strawberries, blackberries, raspberries, are the best choice, as they are rich in nutrients and low in carbohydrates. Adhere to about 1/4 to 1/2 cup per day.

Benefits of a Low-Carbohydrate Diet

1. Rapid Weight Loss

When it comes to losing weight, calorie counting is insane, but in exchange for your attention to the types of foods you eat and focusing on mindful eating can make all the difference. Low carbohydrate diets have a reputation for producing rapid weight loss without feeling hungry or the need to count calories. In fact, many people experience weight loss after a low carb diet, even if they have tried "everything" and never got the results we were looking for.

A 2014 study conducted by the National Institutes of Health found that after comparing the two in overweight adults, low-carb diets were more effective for weight loss and reduced cardiovascular risk factor compared to low-fat diets, as shown by 148 participants of both types of dietary plans over 12 months.

Why are low-carbohydrate diets, especially the keto diet, so effective at shedding excess pounds, even in people who normally struggle to lose weight? When we eat foods with sugar and carbohydrates, the insulin of the hormone is released in a reaction in order to raise the blood glucose (sugar). Insulin is often called "hormone storage fat" because one of your jobs is the cell signal to store as much energy as possible. This energy is stored in the form of glycogen from the glucose found in carbohydrates since glycogen is our "main" energy.

By eliminating carbohydrates from the diet and keeping the body from low or almost empty glycogen stores, we can prevent insulin from being released and storing fat. Less insulin circulating around our bloodstream means that the body is forced to use all of its glycogen stores, then reach the reserves of fat hidden in our adipose tissue (body fat) for the constant fuel.

2. Better Cognitive Function

Fat and carbohydrates tend to have an inverse relationship in the diet. Most people keep their protein intake somewhat stable, but normally the more carbohydrates and sugar that people eat, the less healthy fats they consume. This is problematic because we need healthy fats for proper brain function, mood control and hormonal regulation. Although initially, a sugary or high-carbohydrate meal can make you feel awake and alert, quickly after that it is most likely to break down and you might feel tired, cranky and irritable.

Sugar is addictive and has dramatic effects on the brain, especially when it comes to increased anxiety, anxiety and fatigue. On the other hand, certain types of healthy fats, such as cholesterol, act like antioxidants and precursors to some important brain-supporting molecules and neurotransmitters that control learning, memory,

mood and energy. Your brain is formed largely from fatty acids and requires a constant flow of fats from your diet in order to perform optimally.

Recently, a report published in The Journal of Physiology found evidence of strong metabolic consequences of a high-sugar diet coupled with a deficiency of omega-3 fatty acids on cognitive abilities. These effects are due to the association of the consumption of high amounts of glucose and the action of insulin, which control brain signalling by mediators. As expected, an unhealthy diet that was high in sugar and low in healthy fats such as omega-3 fatty acids is associated with lower cognitive scores and insulin resistance.

The research suggests that the ketogenic diet is especially therapeutic when it comes to protecting cognitive health. The researchers believe that people with the highest insulin resistance could demonstrate less cerebral blood flow and, therefore, less brain plasticity. This is because insulin is a "vasodilator" and increases blood flow to promote the supply of glucose to muscles and organs, including the brain. This vasodilator function stops when someone develops insulin resistance over time from a high sugar content and high carbohydrate intake, resulting in a decrease in brain tissue perfusion and activity.

In some studies, improvement has been observed in Alzheimer's disease and dementia in patients fed a ketogenic diet, marked by factors including improved mitochondrial function. A study noted that new data suggested the therapeutic use of ketogenic diets for several neurological disorders beyond epilepsy and Alzheimer's disease, including headaches, neurotrauma, the disease of Parkinson's, sleep disorders, brain cancer, autism and multiple sclerosis.

3. Reduce the Risk of Metabolic Syndrome and Heart Disease

A study published in The American Journal of Epidemiology found that low-carbohydrate diets are more effective in reducing certain metabolic and heart disease risk factors than low-fat diets are, in addition to at least equal of effective in reducing weight and other factors.

The study investigated the effects of low-carbohydrate diets (45 per cent of energy from carbohydrates) compared to low-fat diets (30 per cent of fat energy) of risk factors metabolic by performing a meta-analysis of randomized controlled trials. Twenty-three trials from several countries, with a total of 2,788 participants were included in the analysis.

The results showed that both low carb and low-fat diets lose weight and improved metabolic risk factors. But, compared to participants about low-fat diets, people on low-carbohydrate diets experienced a significantly greater increase in "good" (high-density lipoprotein cholesterol and a greater decrease in triglyceride levels.

They also experienced a lower reduction in total cholesterol and low-density lipoprotein cholesterol than the low-fat diet group. However, keep in mind that the increase in cholesterol levels has not been shown to contribute to heart disease!

These findings were true, despite the fact that reductions in body weight, waist circumference and other metabolic risk factors were not significantly different between the two groups of diets. These findings suggest that satisfying low carb diets, which are higher in fat, can help fight heart disease factors, as well as diets that are harder to adjust and prone to leaving people hungry.

4. Lower Risk of Type 2 Diabetes

The researchers note that despite the rising rate of type 1 and 2 diabetes and the acceleration of the cost of resources needed to control and treat diabetic patients, the medical community, in general, has not succeeded in reducing the number of people affected or the severity of the complications. While diabetes medication prescriptions continue to rise, there is a simple, effective and inexpensive strategy that is proven to work with diabetes: Reduce the amount of sugar and starch in the diet.

Researchers from the Division of Endocrinology, Diabetes and Hypertension at SUNY of the University of Brooklyn point out that a diet high in carbohydrates elevates plasma postprandial glucose and insulin secretion, which increases the risk of diabetes, heart disease, hypertension, dyslipidemia and obesity.

Many studies have shown that a diet low in carbohydrates is a natural treatment of diabetes and effective tool in the prevention of patients with type 2 diabetes. It can also help to reduce the risk of complications of diabetes and associated risk factors like obesity or heart disease.

A growing body of evidence shows that despite a diet high in "healthy carbohydrates" such as whole grains it is recommended that for many sick patients, low carb diets are comparable, if not better than traditional low fat and high carbohydrate diets for weight reduction, dyslipidemia improvement of diabetes and metabolic syndrome, as well as control of blood pressure, postprandial glycemia and insulin secretion.

In a 2005 study published in The Upsala Journal of Medical Science, for the two groups of obese patients with type 2 diabetes, the effect of two different composition diets was tested with respect to glycemic control and body weight. A group of 16 obese patients with type 2 diabetes was put on a low-carbohydrate diet (1,800 calories for men and 1,600 calories for women) consisting of 20 per cent carbohydrates, 30 per cent protein and 50 per cent fat. %.

Fifteen obese patients with diabetes were put on a high-carbohydrate diet to serve as a control group. Your diet consists of the same calories for men and women including approximately 60% carbohydrates, 15% protein and 25% fat. Positive effects on glucose levels are seen very quickly in the group after the low-carb plan. After six months, a marked reduction in body weight of patients on the low carb diet group was also observed, and this was maintained a year later.

5. Help the Fight Against Cancer

Research shows that a diet high in refined carbohydrates and sugar contributes to the damage of free radicals and actually feeds cancer cells, possibly helping them proliferate faster. Because low-carbohydrate diets drastically reduce sugar and lower grain intake and processed foods, it could act as a natural treatment against cancer, causing immunity to improve as oxidative stress goes down.

Studies indicate that carbohydrate intake influences the biology of prostate cancer, as has been shown through mice that have been fed a no-carbohydrate ketogenic diet (NCKD) significantly experiencing tumours smaller and longer survival times of mice fed a Western diet. Mice fed the equivalent of the normal human Western diet had higher serum insulin, which was associated with significantly higher blood glucose and tumour tissue growth.

In the process of cutting off the energy supply of cancer cases, healthy cells luckily preserved, since they are able to use fat as energy. Cancer cells, on the other hand, thrive off glucose and do not metabolically shift to use fat.

6. Fewer Cravings and Not Go Hungry!

One of the greatest benefits of a low carbohydrate diet or keto diet is that eating more healthy fats and proteins instead of sugar and carbohydrates are super satisfying since it effectively helps to deactivate ghrelin, the hunger of the hormone."

According to studies, insulin regulates ghrelin negatively, and high-density lipoproteins can be a carrier of particles to increase the circulation of ghrelin. In other words, peak insulin carbohydrates quickly, leading to cravings for more food, later, as blood sugar drops and ghrelin increases. Fats and proteins, on the other hand, are known by commutation in the body of satiety hormones and allowing you to go more comfortably between meals without needing to sting.

7. Better Digestion

Less sugar means a better digestive function for most people since sugar feeds "bad bacteria" that can grow in the intestine. The result of a diet too high in sugar and carbohydrates can mean the development of candida virus, irritable bowel syndrome and worse of the symptoms of the leaky gut syndrome. A lot of vegetables, quality proteins and healthy fats, on the other hand, can act as the fat burning of foods that also help to nourish the digestive tract and reduce the growth of bacteria.

Research from a 2008 study published in the Journal of the American Gastroenterological Association showed that patients with irritable bowel syndrome (IBS) report improvements in symptoms after the initiation of the very low carbohydrate content of the diet (VLCD). When participants with moderate to severe IBS were provided with two weeks of standard diet, after four weeks of a VLCD (20 grams of carbohydrates per day), most reported improvements in abdominal pain, stool habits and quality of life.

8. Better Hormone Regulation

We have already learned about the positive effects that a low carbohydrate diet can have on insulin and appetite hormones, but going low in carbohydrates also seems to help balance the function of the neurotransmitter in some people and thus improve mood.

When researchers from the Discipline of Psychiatry and the School of Medicine at the University of Adelaide, compared to the hormonal and psychological effects of a low protein, high carbohydrate (LPHC) and high protein diet, low Carbohydrate (HPLC) diet in women with a hormonal disorder called polycystic ovarian syndrome (PCOS) over the course of 16 weeks, found a significant reduction in depression and improved self-esteem in those who diet low in carbohydrates.

All participants attended a weekly exercise, support group and educational program and completed the Anxiety and Depression Scale Hospital at the beginning and end of the study. The HPLC diet appeared to help balance hormones naturally and was associated with significant reductions in several of the depressive symptoms, improve feelings of well-being and a greater likelihood of having the best long-term adherence to obesity treatment.

Precautions when starting a Low-Carbohydrate Diet

In general, there seems to be a lot of variabilities when it comes to how low-carbohydrate diet and changes in mood and energy levels - with some people feeling good and others struggling a bit at first. Therefore, it is important to pay attention to how it feels to change your diet and make the necessary adjustments.

Self-reports, along with data from certain tests, indicate that too low in carbohydrates, diet or ketogenic diets could increase symptoms such as fatigue, constipation, brain fog and irritability in some people - side effects that They have been dubbed "the carb of influenza" or "flu keto ." However, this is usually the case when you cut carbohydrates drastically to only about 5 per cent to 10 per cent of your total calories. These side effects usually disappear within 1-2 weeks of changing your diet, after your body adapts.

Obviously, the reduction in the desire to be physically active, experiencing brain fog and being in a bad mood is quite counterproductive for people looking to feel healthier and lose weight, so these effects are something to control themselves same. If you feel very slow, in a bad mood, or as if you had «brain fog» and can not think clearly, while after the drastic reduction of carbohydrates over the course of several weeks, especially if you have changed your Diet quickly and carbohydrate reduction very low ketogenic levels to try the reintroduction of some carbohydrates several days a week until you feel better. Experiencing the benefits of low carb diets can take a bit of trial and error.

Final Thoughts on Low Diets in Carbohydrates:

✓ A low-carbohydrate diet is a diet that limits carbohydrates - such as foods with added sugar, grains, starchy vegetables, and fruits - and emphasizes foods high in protein and fat.

✓ Benefits of low carbohydrate diets include help with weight loss, reduction of hunger, better control of insulin and blood sugar, improved cognitive performance, lower risk of heart disease, factors of the improvement of neurological health, and the reduction of the risk of certain types of cancer.

✓ Low-carbohydrate diets tend to be very high in fat or high in protein. A very high-fat content, low carb diet is called the ketogenic diet. This diet causes the body to create ketones and burn fat as fuel, which has many benefits.

✓ On most low-carb diets, you get about 30 per cent or less of your daily carbohydrate calories. Keto diets involve getting 75 per cent or more of the calories coming from the fat, while high protein diets generally involve obtaining 30 per cent or more of the calories from the protein.

✓ Low-carbohydrate diets or ketogenic diets may increase symptoms such as fatigue, constipation, brain fog and irritability in some people. These side effects usually disappear within 1-2 weeks, although some people will ultimately feel better eating at a more moderate carbohydrate position.

CHAPTER 05

KETO DIET AND INTERMITTENT FASTING

Intermittent fasting and the ketogenic diet are two of the main trends in diet patterns and the health of fans. However, while there are a lot of differences between intermittent fasting vs. keto, they can actually be combined to help amplify the results and get to ketosis even faster. In fact, by practising intermittent fasting in keto, you can take advantage of the unique benefits they have to offer.

Why should I fast in keto? What ingredients are found in the diet keto food list? And how many hours should intermittent fasting? Here is everything you need to know about intermittent fasting in keto, as well as how to start.

Why is Intermittent Fasting and keto are Recommended?

Intermittent fasting is a technique that involves restricting food intake for a certain window of time each day and then fasting for a specific period. There are several different fasting methods, with many variations that can be adapted to almost any personal or routine preference. Some of the most common types of intermittent fasting include two days of fasting, fasting 16/8 and diet 5: 2, each of which varies depending on the amount of time you spend fasting during the week.

Fasting in keto can be very beneficial, especially if you have reached a plateau and do not see the results of the ketogenic diet alone. Although it is not necessary, keto intermittent fasting can bring the benefits of diet to the next level and help optimize your health. It is also thought to accelerate ketosis, helping the body to burn glycogen stores more quickly, which can help bypass the symptoms of flu keto for faster results.

There are a lot of keto and intermittent fasting success stories, and hence several reasons you may wish to consider adding to your routine. In particular, keto fasting has been associated with several benefits, including:

✓ Improves Heart Health: According to a study published in the journal PLoS One, fasting is effective in improving cholesterol levels, which could potentially help reduce the risk of heart disease.

✓ Increasing Weight Loss: Studies show that fasting can reduce body weight and body fat while also helping to preserve muscle mass to improve body composition.

✓ Better Control of Blood Sugar: Not only can fast lower blood sugar levels, but it can also increase insulin sensitivity to help your body use insulin more efficiently.

✓ Decreased Inflammation: Several studies have found that fasting can reduce several inflammatory markers, which are thought to play a central role in health and immune function.

✓ Reduce Hunger: Fasting Intermittent keto could decrease the levels of leptin, the satiety hormone that signals your brain when it is time to stop eating. Keeping leptin levels low can help prevent leptin resistance to help keep hunger and appetite under control.

✓ Promotes Brain Function: Studies in Animals show that fasting can improve cognitive function and preserve brain health through the specific influence of proteins involved in brain ageing.

How Fast Flashing in keto

For now, you may ask: how can I make keto and intermittent fasting? By following a few simple steps, it is very easy to get started and prepare for success.

1. Choose Your Protocol

There are different fasting protocols, so it is easy to find a method that works for you. To start, just choose a protocol that fits your daily routine and jump right. Here are some of the most common methods:

✓ Alternate Days of Fasting: This type of eating pattern involves fasting on alternate days. On fasting days, you can refrain from eating completely or limit your intake to around 500 calories per day. In the non-fasting days, you should follow a healthy diet keto as usual.

✓ The Fasting 16/8: The 16/8 intermittent fasting ketosis plan involves fasting for 16 hours a day and limiting your food intake for only 8 hours a day. This usually involves not eating anything after dinner and skipping breakfast the next morning.

✓ 5: 2 Diet: In this plan, you follow a standard diet keto for five days of the week and restrict your intake to around 500-600 calories for the remainder of the two days.

✓ 23/1 Intermittent Fasting Ceto: With this method of intermittent fasting, you should limit your food intake to only one hour a day and fast for the other 23 hours a day.

Intermittent fasting and the keto diet are arguably two of the biggest health trends of the moment, and if you are curious about what would happen if you combined the two together, the expert said that they can pair up nicely and may treat your body to numerous health benefits.

2. Calculate Your Keto Macros

After determining your preferred protocol of intermittent fasting, you should begin to plan your diet during the days you eat. On a keto diet, 75 per cent of total calories must come from fats, 20 per cent must be from protein and 5% must come from carbohydrates. When they started, however, you can start with a diet modification keto place, which is often considered more flexible and easy to follow. With this diet plan, about 40 to 60 per cent of the calories should come from healthy fats with 20-30 per cent of the protein in your food and 15 to 25 per cent of carbohydrates.

There are a lot of online calculators that can help determine your daily calorie intake based on factors such as age, gender and activity level. As a general rule, however, men and women need around 2,500 calories and 2,000 calories per day, respectively, to help maintain weight.

3. Make a Meal Plan

Once you have calculated your daily nutrient needs and decided that the fasting method works for you, you can begin to plan your meals to start with intermittent keto and fasting.

Fill your plate with plenty of healthy fats, such as coconut oil, avocados, olive oil, butter and grass-fed butter as well as moderate amounts of protein from foods like grass-fed meat, poultry, fatty fish and the eggs. Non-starchy vegetables, fresh herbs, nuts, seeds and healthy beverages such as water, bone broth and green tea can enjoy everything as well.

4. Start!

Now that you are prepared correctly, it is time to start fasting with intermittent keto. In addition to reducing carbohydrates, increasing your fat intake and restricting your food intake in a specific period of time each day, you should also make sure you stay hydrated and plan your workout routine around your schedule of fasting. While exercise is good during the days that you fast, it is important to listen to your body and avoid straining too much.

So how long does it take to get into ketosis when fasting? On a keto diet, it usually takes about 2-3 days to get to ketosis, although it can take up to seven days in some cases. However, many people find that keto intermittent fasting adaptation can accelerate the process and help your body burn glycogen reserves more quickly to help enter ketosis.

Keto Fasting Precautions

Although intermittent fasting and keto may be safe and effective for most, it may not be suitable for everyone.

For those with low blood sugar, for example, spending long periods without eating can lower blood sugar levels and cause adverse side effects such as weakness, tremors and sweating. Therefore, if you have diabetes, you should check with your doctor to determine if intermittent keto fasting is right for you.

Intermittent keto fasting is also not recommended for children, pregnant women or people with a history of eating disorders. Instead, it is better to focus on a nutrient-rich diet that can help provide the vitamins and minerals that your body needs.

In addition, although many people use intermittent keto fasting for bodybuilding, it is best to listen to your body when it comes to fasting and physical activity. While exercise light is usually fine, it is recommended to limit exercise on an empty stomach for 72 hours or more.

keep in mind that fasting to induce ketosis can also trigger a series of symptoms often referred to as the " flu keto ." Fasting ketosis symptoms can include decreased energy levels, increased anxiety, problems digestive, muscle pain and dizziness. These symptoms can last from a few days to a few weeks at the start of the ketogenic diet, but usually, disappear once your body goes into ketosis, and it begins to adapt.

"Intermittent fasting and keto are actually very complimentary "When paired together, you can expect to crave less junk food, experience fat loss, and experience an energy boost."

You won't, however, want to fast and observe this high-fat eating plan at the same time without taking some precautions.

It's best to start by tackling one before beginning the other

It's important to give yourself plenty of time to begin the keto diet and overcome any initial " keto flu" symptoms before incorporating intermittent fasting into your routine.

If you're doing both diets at the same time, experts recommend fasting for 12 hours, trying the 16:8 method of fasting or doing a long fast

"Start with a shorter fasting window (12 hours) and build upon it once you get into more of a routine and making sure you are getting the right percentage of healthy fat you need in a day.

"A popular combination would be to use a ketogenic diet as a base and to add a 16:8 fasting schedule to your routine. This means fasting for 16 hours of the day and eating a keto diet during an eight-hour eating window.

You can also try eating one meal a day (a 24-hour fast) and using the keto diet as a guide. "This might be done two or three times per week.

If you're wondering how long you should wait, experts say that those with the keto flu will typically experience symptoms for about a week, although some experience it for even longer.

Doing both diets at the same time calls for more planning

The keto diet is focused on getting the right level of macros each day and intermittent fasting is all about reducing the amount of time you consume food each day. Therefore, if you want to incorporate both plans into your everyday life, planning your meals and snacks a little bit more.

WHY KETO IS MORE EFFECTIVE WITH INTERMITTENT FASTING

Boosts fat loss: Eating all your meals in an 8-hour window (say, eating between noon and 8 PM, and fasting the other 16 hours a day) causes significant weight loss without counting calories. While this type of intermittent fasting causes weight loss no matter what people eat, research shows that people who do it in a healthy manner lose twice as much weight (7% vs. 3% of their body weight) as those who fast while still eating junk. So it's still important to follow a high-performance diet like the Bulletproof Diet while you fast.

Increases muscle gain: Worried about losing muscle if you fast? Maybe this will put your concerns to rest: a single 24-hour fast increased human growth hormone (HGH) by 2000% in men and 1300% in women. HGH plays an integral role in building muscle. Boosting your levels this high will have a huge effect on your physique. Research shows that higher levels of HGH lead to lower levels of body fat, higher lean body mass.

Speeds up recovery: HGH also drives muscle protein synthesis, which speeds up repair and helps you recover faster from a hard workout or an injury.

Makes skin supple: HGH lowers naturally as you age. But when subjects were given HGH supplements, not only did lose fat and build muscle, their skin thickness improved — making it stronger and more resilient to sagging and wrinkles

Slows down aging: Fasting ramps up your stem cell production. Stem cells are like biological playdough — your body turns them into any kind of cell it needs and uses them to replace old or damaged cells, keeping you younger on a cellular level. Stem cells are great for your skin, joints, old injuries, chronic pain, and more. You can try stem cell therapy…or you can just fast.

MENTAL TRICKS TO EAT HEALTHIER AND LOSE WEIGHT

These tricks help you cheat your brain to control your portions and better select your food. Over time this difference in calories can help you achieve your ideal weight.

Remember that it is a gradual process, but it is constant (and without rebound), the best of all is that you will be really creating healthy habits in your routine that stay with you forever. In addition, your palate and your brain will adjust to these changes, the healthy food that previously tasted tasteless will start to like you and without realizing you will already be enjoying these healthy options that help you lose weight.

Let's see these psychological tricks!

1.Use smaller plates and longer cups

When you use very large plates, unconsciously you serve larger portions.

Your brain is easily deceived by changes in perspective, something like an optical effect. Using this in your favor, you can slightly reduce the amount of food you eat without feeling deprived. The use of smaller plates is a proven way to eat less and lose weight (without realizing it). Therefore, size does matter when it comes to your plate. But once you have found a reasonable size, an important question appears, what will I serve on that plate? We tend to start thinking about how much meat, chicken, fish or stew we will serve, that is to say, we see protein as the protagonist of our plate, but here comes the trick to lose weight.If we start thinking about vegetables as the protagonists, it is likely that all the food will become healthier automatically.

Now that you know that the size of the glasses is important, the same goes for the glasses ...

You can reduce your liquid calories by choosing taller glasses and not shorter and wider ones. However, although this trick of the glass is effective a better easy rule to memorize to lose weight is the following:

1.DO NOT drink calories.

That is to say, if you are very thirsty, drink water and nothing else.

It has been seen that sugary drinks contribute to weight gain and the onset of diabetes, so drinking a can of soda does not help you lose weight, even if you drink is dietary.

Remember that your brain is easy to cheat and if you consume something that tastes sweet, but does not provide sugar (such as dietary sweeteners) your brain continues with the craving for something sweet and makes you more susceptible to falling into a sugary trap later.

2.Count the number of times you chew your food

Start to do it as a game that helps you taste your food and eat more carefully.

Count the number of times you chew each food (you'll be surprised how little it is). Try to increase the number in each bite. In this way, avoid eating more than the account and you will feel more satisfied without feeling about to explode. What also helps make the decisions after this meal much healthier and lose weight will be a simple task. Besides, eating slowly is a way of thinking about what you have on your plate. It is important to promote a philosophy of respect for our food, and one way to do it is to taste them.

3.Measure your portions before serving and do not eat directly from the container

We have all done it once: go to the fridge and while we think about eating, we start eating the leftovers from the previous day directly from the container or drinking from the container.

But, this is not helping you lose weight.

It has been shown that eating directly from the container, causes us to lose control over the food portions, which makes us eat much more than the amount needed to satisfy us.Therefore, it is important that you always measure what you serve and do not eat directly from the container.

Do you remember the trick of the smaller plates?

You can do the same to fool your brain: use a smaller spoon to serve yourself, so unconsciously you will feel that you are serving much more than usual.

4.Divide the large container into smaller ones

How much chocolate do you need to satisfy your cravings? How many almonds do you need to satisfy your hunger for half a day? ...

According to one study, consuming a larger portion causes you to consume more than 70% of the food and of course more calories, but small, small portions are able to provide a similar feeling of satisfaction as the larger portions. Surely you remember when you were in kindergarten and your lunch always came in small bags. One trick is to do the same: place your food in small plastic bags or small containers. This helps you feel as if you eat the whole package and it satisfies your brain. For example, The bag of nuts (such as walnuts, almonds, pistachios or peanuts) divides it into more small bags. When you feel a craving or hunger between meals, you will only have to take a small bag. An important point, do not eat directly from a package, serve the portion in a container.

5.Place healthy foods in sight

I remember that an aunt said: I always buy fruit and no one eats it, it's only when I pick it up and put it on the table when it disappears. It is so true, our brain chooses those foods more available and if we are careful to have healthy foods ready to eat, we will be deciding better 100% of the time. In one study, more than 200 kitchens were photographed to determine whether the food in the cupboard or refrigerator was in relation to the weight of the homemaker. Women who had breakfast cereals (even if they were "diet") weighed 9 kilos more than their neighbors who did not have box cereals in the kitchen, and in those refrigerators, with soft drinks, women weighed 11 kilos more. The good news? those who had a bowl of fruit on the table weighed about 5 kilos less. Place fruits and vegetables in sight and at your fingertips, and hide all foods that do not help you lose weight, hide them or move them away from your reach. (Come on, you know what they are). It's like playing hide and seek every time you find a food that contributes to your well-being.

Remember that the best reminder of the habit is visual. If it is in sight it is normal and expected to eat it. An important point, if you want to stop battling with yourself, put your willpower to the test only once in the supermarket and do not buy processed foods or scrap. Remember if they are not within your reach, you do not eat them.

6.Display a pause button inside of you

The next time you feel a powerful magnet towards that extra-large ice cream jar, imagine that you have a pause button inside you. Freeze! try to wait a few minutes and before pressing the play button, think again if you are really hungry or if eating that ice cream is a good decision. The most likely thing is that you can decide in time a better option that will help you lose weight. The binges and many unhealthy food choices are impulsive, therefore, have an imaginary pause button can help you control it effectively. Take the test, you just have to put it into practice and you will develop more self-control in automatic.Fruit juice (even natural) is still a bad choice because the fruit has already lost its fiber and the number of sugars that your body absorbs is similar to a soft drink! You do not believe me? note: an orange juice has 1.8 grams of sugar and a cola drink 1.7 grams. The same goes for alcoholic beverages, so be careful with what you drink.

7.Imagine eating before eating

Thinking about eating a bag of sweets makes it more likely that you will eat less when you actually start eating, according to a 2010 study. The key is to think that you eat that food instead of just thinking about it. This has to do with the release of dopamine in your brain. This substance is responsible for the feeling of satisfaction when eating or drinking. For example: think about how good an ice cold glass of water makes you feel on a very hot day when you have not drunk anything for hours. Suddenly, the sensation is associated with intense emotional pleasure, which disappears little by little. This is called habituation and it leads to a decrease in the dopamine response that makes drinking this ice cold cup of water you imagined, less pleasurable. The same can happen with food and sweets. If we visualize ourselves eating a sweet, our bodies produce the same dopamine response, as if we were actually eating sweets. Therefore, when you really have candy available, your emotional response is not as strong and you eat much less, or it becomes much easier to ignore this whim.

The participants of the study that were visualized eating 30 m & m's before enjoying these, they ate less in comparison with the other participants who only imagined the sweets (without eating them)

8.Make your own list of distractions

This can be an alternative plan when the pause button does not work. Having a list of distractions helps you quickly decide what to do to distract yourself and avoid binge eating. You can also have a boat with papers that have written activities when you feel the urge to eat something unhealthy, you just have to take a paper and do what is written. It's like a child's game to lose weight but it works!

The list can include anything: play, talk with a friend, take a walk, read, listen to music, brush your teeth, drink water, wash dishes, check your mail, etc.

CHAPTER 06

WORKOUTS TO LOSE WEIGHT AND TARGET STUBBORN FAT

There are many workouts to lose weight on the market today, maybe too many. Which ones are the most effective to burn through your belly fat? How can you ever hope to see your rock hard abs?

These answers are not new. They aren't unique, not novel, not even "secrets" at this point.

First, you will need to be sure that you follow a total health regimen. You don't want to run roughshod over your health, but you want to ensure that you do take care of yourself overall. This includes:

✓ Getting enough water daily.

✓ Doing what you can to ·naturally enhance your metabolism.

✓ Getting a full night of sleep.

✓ Eating a diet that nourishes and will detox your system.

✓ Getting the proper workout.

The best exercises to lose weight are those where you spend more calories in less time such as running or swimming, but to lose weight efficiently and maintain results it is important to combine these exercises with muscle exercises that must be performed in the gym, preferably under the supervision of a personal trainer.

Aerobic exercises such as walking and running increase the heart rate and burn more calories, while endurance exercises such as muscles favor muscle hypertrophy allowing an increase in muscle size causing the individual to consume more energy.

The best exercises to lose weight in the gym are aerobics, some examples are:

1. Hit training

The hit training helps burn around 400 calories per hour and consists of a set of high-intensity exercises that help eliminate localized fat in just 30 minutes per day, in the fastest and most fun way. The exercises are done intensively to raise the heart rate a lot and, for this reason, this training is more suitable for people who already practice some kind of physical activity. However, there are hit training routines with easier exercises, special for beginners.

2. Crossfit training

The Crossfit training is also quite intense and burns around 700 calories per hour, however, this type of training is quite different from what people are accustomed to doing in the gym. In the exercises to exercise the muscles in the crossfit, different weights, jump ropes, rubbers, boxes, among others are used and, usually, it is usually done in the open air.

3. Dance Classes

Dancing is an excellent way to strengthen muscles and burn calories, 1 hour of ballroom dancing helps burn about 300 calories. In addition to this, depending on the type of dance the person can increase flexibility, improve posture and have fun. In this type of activity in addition to cardiorespiratory and weight loss benefits, socialization is also promoted. Some activities of this kind can also be performed outdoors, as in the case of Zumba or biotherapy, which help burn up to 800 kcal per hour.

4. Muay Thai

Muay Thai is a type of intense martial art, where it is possible to burn around 700 calories per hour. The workouts are quite intense and help strengthen the muscles, in addition to helping to increase self-esteem and teach self-defense

5. Spinning

Spinning classes have different intensities, and it is done in a room with an exercise bike. The classes are usually quite intense and usually burn about 600 calories per hour, helping to strengthen the legs, being excellent for burning fat from the legs and strengthening the thighs and calves.

6. Swimming

In a swimming class, you can burn up to 400 calories per hour, as long as the student does not lose the rhythm and always keep moving. Although the strokes are not very strong to reach the other side of the pool faster, a constant effort is necessary, with a few rest periods. When the goal is to lose weight you should not only reach the other side of the pool, it is necessary to maintain a constant and strong rhythm, that is, you can cross the pool swimming crawl and back, for example, as a way of 'rest' .

7. Hydrogym

Hydro-gymnastics is also excellent for weight loss, but to burn around 500 calories per hour you must always keep moving, enough to be panting.

As water relaxes the tendency is to slow down, however, if you want to lose weight, the ideal is to be in a class whose purpose is the same, because there are classes for older people that are at a slower pace, and in these cases It is not enough to help you lose weight.

8. Running

The race training is excellent for burning fat, being possible to burn around 600 to 700 calories per hour, provided that good rhythm is respected, without pauses, and with enough effort to be panting, unable to converse during the race. You can start at a slower pace, both on the treadmill and in the open air, however, each week you should gradually increase the intensity to achieve the desired goal.

9. Body pump

Body pump classes are an excellent way to burn fat because in 1 hour of class you can burn 500 calories approximately. This is a class made with weights and step, so it helps to work and strengthen the main muscle groups.

HOW TO DETECT KETOSIS

Restricting carbohydrates means less glucose

The body of a healthy person who gets their nutrition from a balanced proportion of macronutrients - protein, carbohydrates and fat - burns glucose as their main source of energy. Glucose usually comes from carbohydrate-based foods (such as bread, pasta, fruits, vegetables, whole grains, soft drinks, etc.). It is used to supply energy to the body or is stored as glycogen in the muscles and liver. When calories or carbohydrates are reduced strictly, there is enough glucose available to the body. As such, the body seeks an alternative strategy to meet its energy demands and continue to function properly.

The state of ketosis: finding an alternative source of energy

The state of ketosis means that the body switched its dependence on carbohydrates as energy by burning fat as fuel. That means not just food fats (olive oil, guacamole, fried pig's ears) but also body fat - clearly a desirable situation for anyone who wants to lose extra weight.

When the body metabolizes fat, it generates molecules called ketones (also known as ketone bodies). As you restrict your intake of carbohydrates and increase dietary fat, more fat is metabolized and a greater amount of ketones is created. Most cells in your body - including those in the brain - are able to use ketone as energy, although many people experience a period of adaptation (1-3 days), commonly called low-carb flu.

For healthy individuals, ketosis usually comes into action after 3 to 4 days of eating less than 50 grams of carbohydrate per day. Ketosis can also occur after a very long exercise session, during pregnancy or for people with uncontrolled diabetes.

How to detect ketosis

Following a low-carb diet with less than 50 grams of carbohydrates, a day does not necessarily mean that your body will switch to ketosis. For example, exercising or eating too much protein can keep you from ketosis. There are different methods to find out if your body has switched to ketosis.

1.Ketone Breath

Acetone is one of three attributes of ketone bodies, produced as by-products when fatty acids are broken down to produce energy in the liver and kidneys. As a result of the released acetone, the smell of breathing changes as it enters ketosis. It can be described as "fruity" or even "metallic" - compared to mature apples. If you realize this happening on your first days of diet change, it may mean that you have entered into ketosis. Brushing, flossing or shaving the tongue does not help to kill bad breath, but it usually decreases after the first few weeks. Acetone can also be detected using a Ketonix device, which measures the concentration of acetate/acetone in respiration. These devices are quite expensive and not always very accurate.

2.Increased thirst and dry mouth

When switching to a ketogenic state, thirst usually increases. The body uses excess glycogen and increases the urge to urinate. Check if you are thirsty, however, it is very inaccurate to find out if you are in ketosis.

As insulin levels decline following a ketogenic diet, the body begins to expel excess sodium and water. To balance the electrolytes, it is recommended to add 2-4 grams of sodium per day to your diet when in a plane with extremely low carbohydrate content.

3.Detecting ketones in the urine

A more accurate way to check for ketosis is to use urine ketone test strips, often known by the Ketostix brand. Strips are inexpensive and help to quickly check ketone levels. If you are in ketosis, the strip will change colour. The strips usually come with a guide to find out how "deep" is the level of ketosis.

Place the tip of the small paper test strip directly through your urine stream (alternatively, collect urine in a clean, dry container and immerse the strip thereafter). Shake off any excess and wait 15 seconds. The colour meaning of Ketostix is in a tonal spectrum that will show in which state of ketosis you are. Here's a quick summary of how to read ketone strips:

✓ If the keto strip changes colour from your original beige - compare the colour with the tab on the side of the package to find out how "deep" your ketosis level is.

✓ Stronger levels of purple usually indicate higher levels of ketones. This does not mean that deep levels are a desirable state. A low to medium level is usually associated with better overall well-being.

Keep in mind that urine ketone levels do not necessarily correspond to blood ketone levels. For example, the concentration of ketones in your urine changes depending on how hydrated you are. Dehydration can result in a false positive. This is likely to happen when testing ketone levels in the morning. On the other hand, drinking lots of water can result in a lower concentration of ketones, ie a false negative.

Ketone Strip Color Scale

This Ketostix colour chart helps you evaluate if ketosis has been reached and, if so, to what extent. Be sure to wait precisely 15 seconds after the test strip comes in contact with the urine and compare the colour of the test area with that of the corresponding spectrum.

4.Blood tests

Blood tests are the most accurate (and most expensive) way to measure if your body has switched to ketosis. Blood ketone testing is usually used by people with diabetes. To test your ketone levels, you need a blood ketone meter and a kit that includes a pen with lancet and ketone test strips. Do not confuse ketone test strips with glucose test strips as they do not test for ketones.

The body is typically in ketosis when the blood ketone meter measures between 0.5 and 3 mml / L.

Potential urine ketone test errors

Urine ketone levels do not necessarily correspond to blood ketone levels. There are a few reasons why this may occur.

Hydration can have a great influence on the concentration of ketones in your urine. Dehydration can result in a false positive, something that some people believe happens every morning in a mild degree. Likewise, drinking a ton of liquids - and you should drink water as if it were your job - will result in a lower concentration of ketones, which means a false negative.

Over time, people following ketogenic diets tend to measure lower levels of ketones in the urine, although they are still solidly in the fat-burning mode. At this point, a blood test may be needed to accurately test ketosis - but these are significantly more expensive (besides, you have to prick your finger rather than simply urinate). If you have been following good eating habits and consistently have been on ketosis in the weeks that follow, there is probably no need to worry about it.

CHAPTER 07

AUTOPHAGY AS A NATURAL DETOXIFICATION PROCESS OF THE BODY

HISTORY IN BRIEF

Autophagy is a process of "self-consumption" in which your body digests damaged cells. It is a cleansing process that encourages the proliferation of new and healthy cells

The cyclicity of nutrition is a crucial factor in promoting health. Cells are produced or detoxified, and each phase has its own requirements

Cyclic ketosis and intermittent fasting inhibit inflammation in the body and activate the process of autophagy, a natural process that cleanses and detoxifies cells and recycles the parts of organelles that are no longer needed

To activate the process of autophagy, whether you fast or not fast, you must first consume fats and then carbohydrates. Also, you should include more foods that stimulate such a process, such as citrus bergamot tea, turmeric and green tea

Cyclic exercise-that is, doing 30 minutes of training at high-intensity intervals or resistance training every other day-also helps activate and deactivate the autophagy process.

Autophagy is the natural process by which our body removes out cellular junk to let new cell growth. It makes total sense that our body needs an internal clean up to detox and repairs itself. Autophagy destroys parts of the cell, proteins and cell membranes which are not functioning properly.

How Autophagy Works

It is a biological process, where the key players are tiny cells called lysosomes, which contain enzymes needed to digest and breakdown parts of the cell that no longer function properly. That said, there is a dangerous side because lysosomes are very effective and a prolonged state of autophagy can lead to cell death, a process called autolysis. So a certain amount of autophagy is good, but too much can be damaging to our health.

Why this Cellular Junk Removal Process is so necessary

Our body needs to regularly clean out any junk that is lying around in our cells, or else our cells become less efficient and deteriorate. When our cells are not working properly, our body becomes more sensitive to degeneration. Autophagy makes our bodies more efficient, stops cancerous growth and metabolic dysfunction like diabetes and obesity.

How autophagy affects our cells

With it, we keep our cells healthy. Our cells need cleaning from ineffective parts to avoid an imbalance between free radical damage and the antioxidants needed to prevent it. Without it, our body will experience inflammation caused by oxidative stress. It is also necessary to keep muscle strength as you age. By removing cellular junk your muscle stem cells continue to repair your tissues. This is the main reason detox is so important for older athletes.

Some of the benefits of autophagy

✓ Eliminates toxins

✓ Stimulates the immune system

✓ Longevity, favoring the activity of DNA and therefore preventing a multitude of diseases

✓ Favors degenerative disorders such as Alzheimer's and Parkinson's

✓ Regulates inflammation

✓ Prevents type 2 diabetes

Ways to activate autophagy

So how could you activate the autophagy mechanism in your body?

1. Intermittent fasting in combination with a protein cycle (IFPC, for its acronym in English).

Fast intermittently every other day (you should not eat for 16 hours, which is the time needed to activate the autophagy process and you should schedule your feeding in 8 hours). On days when you do not perform intermittent fasting, consume the regular amount of protein you would normally eat, and during the day you perform intermittent fasting, decrease the amount of protein to around 5% of your calories.

" So, for someone who normally consumes between 45 and 50 grams of protein ... [on days of low protein consumption], about 5% of my total caloric intake, which is about 25 grams of protein, "explains Whittel.

2. Nutrient programming. First, consume fats, and then carbohydrates, whether fasting or not intermittently. " In a day of low consumption [of protein], when you have done an intermittent fast, your first meal should

consist of fats; That must be the first thing I eat. Then, at the end of the day, you can consume carbohydrates, but we refer to the quality carbohydrates we need to be healthy.

Also, when you consume carbohydrates at night as your last meal, you will reap the benefits, from stimulating recovery to helping you relax and getting ready for sleep. Therefore, my second principle is that you must first consume fats and then carbohydrates, "says Whittel.

3. Cyclic exercise. Every two days, you should do 30 minutes of training at high-intensity intervals or resistance training. "It could be as simple as walking faster for a minute and then slowing down, and doing that back and forth for 30 minutes.

Even resistance training could consist of doing yoga, "he says." That acute stress that causes, is an excellent type of stress, which generates a beneficial effect on autophagy. "

4. Eat more foods that activate the autophagy process. Whittel includes 140 different types of foods that help activate the process of autophagy - such as citrus bergamot tea, turmeric and green tea - and others that are recommended depending on whether or not that day intermittently fasts and implements a low protein consumption

For example, on a fast day, with low protein consumption, it is recommended to eliminate egg white (the part with a high protein content) when eating eggs. On days when you do not fast or eat a lot of protein, you should eat both the egg white and the egg yolk.

Intermittent fasting: Autophagy is activated when we put our body under mild stress.

Exercise: With exercise, we activate the detox of our body and cellular renewal. When you exercise your body experiences mild stress, which promotes growth and activates the process.

Ketosis: A low carbohydrate diet induces Ketosis, a state when our liver produces ketones which become the primary fuel for our body. This process activated autophagy which sends the signal to our body to start cleaning our cells. Our health depends on our healthy cells, that is why our body uses autophagy to revitalize our cells. You can also take supplements to support your body at the cellular level and improve its function.

Exercise is the most common and effective way to activate autophagy, but they must be of high intensity, such as HIIT training of high intensity, tabatas, or in the case of exercises with weights, use rest pause or descending systems, since autophagy is closely related to the AMPK energy system, and these systems are the ones that benefit the most in this case.

The intermittent fasting is the best way to induce autophagy , when we fast we force the body to self clean, and begins to consume other components such as cellular food, grease and debris, leaving smartly aside the necessary and burning unnecessary first as waste and persistent toxins.

Diets such as ketogenic or hybrid diet are the systems that offer the most benefits on autophagy and longevity demonstrated by the medical and scientific community, and without the need to be fasting.

There are many types of fasting, but in this case the important thing is to fast more than the usual 8 hours of minimum sleep, this can be done simply by skipping breakfast or postponing it a few hours later, although there are many who go beyond fasting 12 / 12h, 16 / 8h, or even 24h. In the case of strength sports or hypertrophy, where catabolism can make us lose muscle mass, it is not advisable to fast more than 12h (as long as we talk about natural athletes), and in the case of wanting to do so I recommend including 5g (no more takes) of essential amino acids in free form every 3-4h.

The supplementation is another way of inducing autophagy, although indirectly makes the brain into believing that fasting is under even exercise. This is achieved by raising the metabolic pathway ampk, the most common are: coffee, green tea, Resveratrol, alpha lipoic acid, etc.

CHAPTER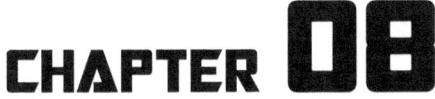

HOW TO COUNT MACROS IN YOUR DIET

What are macros?

In order not to get too caught up, I'll summarize it in this: protein, carbohydrates, fat, and alcohol.

PROTEIN

Apart from everything you already know about tissue repair and the creation/maintenance of muscle, protein helps us control our appetite in different ways. The digestion of the protein needs much more energy than the rest of macros (your body burns more to digest it) and makes you feel fuller for longer as that process of digestion is also slower.

That is why it is normal to hear that high protein diets are usually effective when losing fat. What you must understand is that you tend to eat fewer calories in general because you are full, there is nothing magical about eating protein but it is essential for our health.

Where do we find it?

Meat, fish, eggs, and dairy are good examples. You may have heard about other sources of protein such as nuts and legumes, and although 15% of all calories from these foods come from protein, having them as the main sources of protein would not be very successful.

If we put the almonds as an example, we are talking about a composition of 75% fat and 15% protein; This does not mean that you should not eat almonds, it is simply for you to get used to the idea that "nuts are a good source of protein" does not make much sense.

How much do I need?

There are a thousand ways to calculate it and it depends on several factors, but if improving your physique is the goal, between 2 - 2.3g per kg of weight would be a starting point.

CARBOHYDRATES

What do they do?

Our body uses carbohydrates as energy. They are stored in the liver, brain, blood, and muscles as glycogen. They also make the food creak and get richer as a rule.

Where do we find them?

Fruits, vegetables, rice, bread, cereals, energy drinks / sweetened and a lot of things that you always missed obsessively if you tried a diet low in carbohydrates.

Yes, I've been there, I do not eat a piece of bread because I think it's fattening, it's not cool.

How many do I need?

It also depends. Technically, we can live with 0 carbos but the range is super wide; Bodybuilders or runners consume up to 600 or more grams a day depending on their needs. As usual with everything, you must find the amount you need for your lifestyle and goal. A good start would be between 1.25g per kg of lean mass reaching up to 6-7g + per kg.

GREASES

Fat is an essential nutrient; it helps us with the absorption of vitamins, regulates our hormones, brain functions, etc ... You need to eat fat.

All the fat that we eat is used as energy or accumulates. That does NOT mean that fat, the total calories of the day, week, month, a year is what will make you save that fat more permanently or not. I repeat it again. The fat is NOT bad or fat. We need it to function properly and it gives an incredible flavor to the food!

Where do we find it?

Meat and fatty fish, whole eggs, nuts, oils and butter, cheeses, etc ...

How much do I need?

If you have read the previous sections, you have surely guessed this answer. Exactly, it depends on several things - about 15-45% of your total calories. The total calories that you have an objective will be those that dictate the amount of fat that you eat, try not to lose the total of 15% for that of the hormones and other little things.

ALCOHOL

It may make you more sociable, fun and even noisy. You will have more confidence in yourself (or less), better or worse sex, you may feel euphoric or depressed.It all depends on how much you drink, who you are with and who you are. Being a little more serious, alcohol is not essential nutrient nor is it necessary for anybody function but it gives us calories and that is why we include it as the macro room.

Where do we find it?

Beer, wine, liquors ... Surely you do not need a detailed list, we all know perfectly where it is.

CHAPTER 09

KETO DIET FOOD LIST

Unlike many fad diets that come and go with very limited rates of long-term success, the ketogenic diet (or keto diet) has been practised for more than nine decades (since the 1920s) and is based upon a solid understanding of physiology and nutrition science.

The keto diet works for such a high percentage of people because it targets several keys, underlying causes of weight gain — including hormonal imbalances, especially insulin resistance coupled with high blood sugar levels, and the cycle of restricting and "binging" on empty calories due to hunger that so many dieters struggle with. Yet that's not a problem with what's on the keto diet food list.

What is the keto diet? Rather than relying on counting calories, limiting portion sizes, resorting to extreme exercise or requiring lots of willpower (even in the face of drastically low energy levels), the ketogenic, low-carb diet takes an entirely different approach to weight loss and health improvements. It works because it changes the very "fuel source" that the body uses to stay energized: namely, from burning glucose (or sugar) to dietary fat, courtesy of keto recipes and the ketogenic diet food list items, including high-fat, low-carb diet foods.

Making that switch will place your body in a state of "ketosis," when your body becomes a fat burner rather than a sugar burner. The steps are surprising simple:

✓ Cut down on carbs.

✓ Increase your consumption of healthy fats.

✓ Without glucose coursing through your body, it's now forced to burn fat and produce ketones instead.

✓ Once the blood levels of ketones rise to a certain point, you officially enter into ketosis.

✓ This state results inconsistent, fairly quick weight loss until your body reaches a healthy and stable weight.

Keto Diet Food List, Including the Best Keto Foods

If you're new to the keto diet or just still learning the ropes, your biggest questions probably revolve around figuring out just what high-fat low-carb foods you can eat on such a low-carb, ketogenic diet. Overall, remember that the bulk of calories on the keto diet are from foods that are high in natural fats along with a moderate amount of foods with protein.

Those that are severely restricted are all foods that provide lots of carbs, even kinds that are normally thought of as "healthy," like whole grains, for example.

The biggest shifts in your daily habits will be how your food shop and how you cook, and recipes that are a ketogenic need to be followed rather than just low-carb. You will require healthy fats in order to get into ketosis and have enough energy without carbs. And you will be considerably more energetic and healthier when cooking your own keto-friendly food rather than buying supposedly keto foods off the shelf. So visit my page on keto recipes as well as keto snacks (including fat bombs!), and get started on a ketogenic meal plan!

OVERVIEW OF THE KETO DIET PLAN:

✓ The exact ratio of recommended macronutrients in your diet (grams of carbs vs. fat vs. protein) will differ depending on your specific goals and current state of health. Your age, gender, level of activity and current body composition can also play a role in determining your carb versus fat intake.

✓ Historically, ketogenic diets have consisted of limiting carbohydrate intake to just 20–30 net grams per day. "Net carbs" is the number of carbs remaining once dietary fibre is taken into account. Because fibre is indigestible once eaten, most people don't count grams of fibre toward their daily carb allotment. In other words, total carbs – grams of fibre = net carbs. That's the carb counts that matter most.

✓ On a "strict" (standard) keto diet, fats typically provides about 70 per cent to 80 per cent of total daily calories, protein about 15 per cent to 20 per cent, and carbohydrates just around 5 per cent. However, a more "moderate" approach to the keto diet is also a good option for many people that can allow for an easier transition into very low-carb eating and more flexibility (more on this type of plan below).

✓ Something that makes the keto diet different from other low-carb diets is that it does not "protein-load." Protein is not as big a part of the diet as fat is. Reason being: In small amounts, the body can change protein to glucose, which means if you eat too much of it, especially while in the beginning stages of the keto diet, it will slow down your body's transition into ketosis.

✓ Protein intake should be between one and 1.5 grams per kilogram of your ideal body weight. To convert pounds to kilograms, divide your ideal weight by 2.2. For example, a woman who weighs 150 pounds (68 kilograms) should get about 68–102 grams of protein daily.

✓ It's important to also drink lots of water. Getting enough water helps keep you from feeling fatigued, is important for digestion and aids in hunger suppression.

It's also needed for detoxification. Aim to drink 10–12 eight-ounce glasses a day.

BEST KETO FOODS

Healthy Fats

Most healthy fats contain zero net carbs, especially the kinds listed below, which also have other health advantages. (17) Fats should be included in high amounts with every meal throughout the day.

- ✓ Healthy fats include saturated fats, monounsaturated fats and certain types of polyunsaturated fats (PUFAs), especially omega-3 fatty acids. It's best to include all types in your diet, with an emphasis on saturated fats, especially compared to PUFAs.

- ✓ MCT oil, cold-pressed coconut, palm fruit, olive oil, flaxseed, macadamia and avocado oil — 0 net carbs per tablespoon

- ✓ Butter and ghee — 0 net carbs per tablespoon

- ✓ Lard, chicken fat or duck fat — 0 net carbs per tablespoon

Proteins

Animal proteins (meat, fish, etc.) have very little, if any, carbs. You can consume them in moderate amounts as needed to control hunger. Overall, choose fattier cuts of meat rather than leaner ones. For example, chicken thighs and legs are preferable to chicken breasts because they contain much more fat.

✓ Grass-fed beef and other types of fatty cuts of meat, including lamb, goat, veal, venison and other game. Grass-fed, fatty meat is preferable because it's higher in quality omega-3 fats — 0 grams net carbs per 5 ounces

✓ Organ meats including liver — around 3 grams net carbs per 5 ounces

✓ Poultry, including turkey, chicken, quail, pheasant, hen, goose, duck — 0 grams net carbs per 5 ounces

✓ Cage-free eggs and egg yolks — 1 gram net carb each

✓ Fish, including tuna, trout, anchovies, bass, flounder, mackerel, salmon, sardines, etc. — 0 grams net carbs per 5 ounces

Non-Starchy Vegetables

✓ All leafy greens, including dandelion or beet greens, collards, mustard, turnip, arugula, chicory, endive, escarole, fennel, radicchio, romaine, sorrel, spinach, kale, chard, etc. — range from 0.5–5 net carbs per 1 cup

✓ Cruciferous veggies like broccoli, cabbage, Brussels sprouts and cauliflower — 3–6 grams net carbs per 1 cup

✓ Celery, cucumber, zucchini, chives and leeks — 2–4 grams net carbs per 1 cup

✓ Fresh herbs — close to 0 grams net carbs per 1–2 tablespoons

✓ Veggies that are slightly higher in carbs (but still low all things considered) include asparagus, mushrooms, bamboo shoots, bean sprouts, bell pepper, sugar snap peas, water chestnuts, radishes, jicama, green beans, wax beans, tomatoes — 3–7 grams net carbs per 1 cup raw

Fat-Based Fruit

✓ Avocado — 3.7 grams net carbs per half

Snacks

✓ Bone broth (homemade or protein powder) — 0 grams net carbs per serving

✓ Beef or turkey jerky — 0 grams net carbs

✓ Hard-boiled eggs — 1 gram net carb

- ✓ Extra veggies (raw or cooked) with homemade dressing — 0–5 grams net carbs

- ✓ 1/2 avocado with sliced lox (salmon) — 3–4 grams net carbs

- ✓ Minced meat wrapped in lettuce — 0-1 grams net carbs

Condiments

- ✓ Spices and herbs — 0 grams net carbs

- ✓ Hot sauce (no sweetener) — 0 grams net carbs

- ✓ Apple cider vinegar — 0–1 gram net carbs

- ✓ Unsweetened mustards — 0–1 gram net carbs

Drinks

- ✓ Water — 0 grams of net carbs

- ✓ Unsweetened coffee (black) and tea; drink in moderation since high amounts can impact blood sugar — 0 grams net carbs

- ✓ Bone broth — 0 grams net carbs

Keto Foods To Limit

Eat Only Occasionally:

Full-Fat Dairy

Dairy products should be limited to only "now and then" due to containing natural sugars. Higher fat, hard cheeses have the least carbs, while low-fat milk and soft cheeses have much more.

✓ Full-fat cow's and goat milk (ideally organic and raw) — 11–12 net grams per one cup serving

✓ Full-fat cheeses — 0.5–1.5 net grams per one ounce or about 1/4 cup

Medium-Starchy Vegetables

✓ Sweet peas, artichokes, okra, carrots, beets and parsnips — about 7–14 net grams per 1/2 cup cooked

✓ Yams and potatoes (white, red, sweet, etc.) — sweet potatoes have the least carbs, about 10 net grams per 1/2 potato; Yams and white potatoes can have much more, about 13–25 net grams per 1/2 potato/yam cooked

Legumes and Beans

✓ Chickpeas, kidney, lima, black, brown, lentils, hummus, etc. — about 12–13 net grams per 1/2 cup serving cooked

✓ Soy products, including tofu, edamame, tempeh — these foods can vary in carbohydrates substantially, so read labels carefully; soybeans are fewer in carbs than most other beans, with only about 1–3 net carbs per 1/2 cup serving cooked

Nuts and Seeds

✓ Almonds, walnuts, cashews, sunflower seeds, pistachios, chestnuts, pumpkin seeds, etc. — 1.5–4 grams net carbs per 1 ounce; cashews are the highest in carbs, around 7 net grams per ounce

✓ Nut butter and seed butter — 4 net carbs per 2 tablespoons

✓ Chia seeds and flaxseeds — around 1–2 grams net carbs per 2 tablespoons

Fruits

✓ Berries, including blueberries, strawberries, blackberries, raspberries — 3–9 grams net carbs per 1/2 cup

Snacks

✓ Protein smoothie (stirred into almond milk or water)

✓ 7–10 olives

✓ 1 tablespoon nut butter or a handful of nuts

✓ Veggies with melted cheese

Condiments

Most condiments below range from 0.5–2 net grams per 1–2 tablespoon serving. Check ingredient labels to make sure added sugar is not included, which will increase net carbs. (Stevia and erythritol will become your go-to sweeteners because neither raise your blood sugar — combine for a more natural sweet taste and, remember, a little goes a long way!)

✓ No sugar added ketchup or salsa

✓ Sour cream

✓ Mustard, hot sauces, Worcestershire sauce

✓ Lemon/ lime juice

✓ Soy sauce

✓ Salad dressing (ideal to make your own with vinegar, oil and spices)

✓ Pickles

✓ Stevia (natural sweetener, zero calories and no sugar)

✓ Erythritol

Drinks

Consume the unsweetened drinks below only moderately, having just 1–2 small servings per day. These will typically contain between 1–7 net grams per serving.

✓ Fresh vegetable and fruit juices — homemade is best to limit sugar; use little fruit to reduce sugar and aim for 8 ounces daily at most

✓ Unsweetened coconut or almond milk (ideal to make your own)

✓ Bouillon or light broth (this is helpful with electrolyte maintenance)

✓ Water with lemon and lime juice.

CHAPTER 10

KETO RECIPES HIGH IN HEALTHY FATS LOW IN CARBS

Trying new diets can be tough: all those things to avoid, to eat more of, new ingredients to buy. It's enough to drive anyone bonkers. But there's one way of eating that's been gaining momentum lately — the ketogenic, or "keto," diet and its keto recipes.

The keto diet is one of the most effective that I've come across and one of the more straightforward (as opposed to easy!) to follow. In a nutshell, when you're on a keto diet, you eat a very low-carb, high-fat diet. That means goodbye pasta and bread, hello cheese and oils. It's pretty much the opposite of what we've been taught our entire lives. But it works if you follow the keto diet food list. Plus, you can make many favourite recipes keto-friendly.

What makes the keto diet work so well is that, with little glucose from carbohydrates in our bodies, we have to burn something else — fat — for energy. The keto diet can cause the body to burn fat quite quickly (hurray!).

But even if you're not trying to lose weight, the keto meal plans might appeal to you. By limiting sugars and processed grains, you lower your risk of type 2 diabetes. Eating an array of heart-healthy fats, like nuts, olive oil and fish, can decrease your risk of heart disease. And while some people stick to a super strict keto diet, with 75 per cent of their diet coming from fat, 20 per cent from protein and just five from carbs, even a less intense, modified version can help you reap the keto diet's benefits.

Eating keto doesn't mean eating just any kind of fat or stuffing your face with ice cream. Instead, it's about mindfully choosing foods that are high in healthy fats and low in carbs. If you're not sure where to begin, have no fear. There are some really delicious, good-for-you keto recipes out there that are begging to be eaten.

1. Avocado Deviled Eggs

On the keto diet, sometimes you fall into a pattern of eating a lot of cheese and other dairy products like sour cream and mayonnaise to get all of your necessary daily fats. This avocado deviled eggs recipe gives you the nutrients you need without the dairy for a nice change in the pattern.

2. Chocolate Fat Bombs

The beauty about the keto diet is that sometimes you just haven't eaten enough fat in the day, and so you chow down on "fat bombs" to make up the deficit. These chocolate bombs are one of the yummiest ways to do that. Just mix butter, cream cheese, cocoa powder and a small amount of sweetener for some chocolatey goodness that'll do your body good.

3.Cauliflower Crusted Grilled Cheese Sandwiches

Get a load of veggies and cheese with this ingenious keto recipe. You'll dry out the cauliflower, then bake it into "bread" slices that get stacked with cheese; use a high-quality, organic cheddar here. It's worth it!

4. Chicken Pad Thai

This low-carb chicken pad thai is one of the best keto recipes for replacing Asian takeout. It's got all of the flavours that come with normal pad thai, like ginger, crushed peanuts, tamari and chicken, but all served up on spiralized zucchini instead of carb-heavy noodles. Best of all, you'll have this keto chicken recipe on the table in just 30 minutes.

5. Keto Bread

Bread probably isn't the first thing that comes to mind when you think about the ketogenic diet because it's generally full of carbs. But, if you replace your store-bought bread with a homemade keto bread recipe, it can fit seamlessly into your keto low-carb, high-fat diet. How does bread even become keto-friendly? With almond flour, a lot of eggs, cream of tartar, butter, baking soda and apple cider vinegar.

6. Cinnamon Butter Bombs

Grass-fed butter is a terrific way to add quality fat into your diet. Plus, it's full of health benefits: this type of butter is anti-inflammatory, better for your heart than standard butter and full of MCTs, which boost your immune system.

But if you're not ready to eat a stick of butter solo, just make these cinnamon bombs. By simply adding vanilla extract, cinnamon and keto friendly sweetener to your butter and letting them cool, you have a little treat that's full of healthy fats and tastes like frosting.

7. Coconut Oil Mayonnaise

You'll often find keto recipes calling for mayonnaise. But why waste your money on store-bought varieties that are filled with ingredients like canola oil when you can make your own at home? You'll be surprised by how easy mayo is to whip up at home, and it lasts until your eggs expire!

8. Creamy Cauliflower Mash and Keto Gravy

Potatoes and gravy are total comfort food — and luckily, there's a keto version. These are made with cauliflower, which is quite low-carb, particularly when compared to potatoes. Made with cream, butter, rosemary and parmesan, this mash is creamy, full of flavour and smooth. You'll finish it all off with a stock-based gravy, that would be perfect on a roast, too.

9. Crustless Spinach Quiche

Fortunately, keto recipes can also include quiche. This one looks fancy, but it's effortless to put together. With just a handful of ingredients, including high-protein eggs, lots of cheese and zero grains, it's one of my favourite keto recipes to serve for brunch.

10. Low-Carb Keto Everything Bagels

When you've eaten all of the crustless spinach quiche and keto frittata recipes that you can, these keto everything bagels are another great breakfast staple. With their help, you don't have to cut out your favourite breakfast sandwiches. You can also try a bread-less keto breakfast sandwich with chicken sausage patties as the "buns" when you're craving a keto-approved breakfast option.

11. Simple Paleo Chicken Curry

This coconut chicken curry recipe seems to fit whatever diet you're on because it's gluten-free, dairy-free and uses only the cleanest of ingredients. So, whether you're following the Paleo diet, ketogenic diet or both, this recipe fits your needs. Plus, it's so simple and easy to make.

12. Fathead Nachos

Keto recipes that include nachos?! Oh yes. You'll begin by making the fat head tortilla chips first. Did I mention you'll use two types of cheese for this step? Delicious. Next, you'll load them up with a meaty sauce and finish them off with your favourite toppings, like guac, salsa or sour cream. While these make a delicious keto snack, they're frankly filling enough to share as a meal.

13. Gluten-Free Cauliflower Mac and Cheese

Can you really make a gluten-free, low-carb macaroni and cheese that tastes good? The verdict after trying this keto recipe is yes! Cauliflower, that magical vegetable, stands in for macaroni here, but it's really the cheese and kefir that make this one stand out.

Kefir is a fermented milk-like keto friendly drink that's rich in probiotics and great for your gut. We'll also use sheep and goat milk cheese, which is a smart option for people who are lactose intolerant or just want to vary up their cheese. You'll love serving this, and your family will love eating it.

14. Jalapeño Cheddar Burgers

Why top a burger with cheese when you can stuff it instead? You'll envelop each patty (your choice of turkey or beef) with a mixture of cheeses, garlic and jalapeño, then grill or broil to perfection. Each bite is better than the last.

15. Keto Lime Creamsicles

Most popsicles and ice creams have too much sugar to fall under the category of ketogenic, but these popsicles, sweetened with stevia, can help curb your sweet tooth while giving you a little bit of fat from mashed avocado.

16. Onion Soup

Ditch the canned soup and try this flavorful onion soup recipe filled with powerful nutrients from incorporating both chicken and beef bone broth. This recipe only requires five ingredients total and is quick and simple to throw together. You'll wonder why you ever picked up canned soup in the first place!

17. Keto Spinach and Artichoke Chicken

This juicy chicken has so many rich, delicious flavours happening at once that your taste buds will get a workout. You'll mix spinach, artichokes, garlic, cream cheese, mayo and two types of cheese into a creamy paste, spread it all over the chicken and bake. Bubbly, cheesy goodness awaits after just 40 minutes, with little hands-on time.

18. Keto Grilled Chicken and Spinach Pizza

For a complete keto recipes list, we must include pizza and this is the ultimate keto white pizza. It's got a crisp crust, white sauce, juicy chicken and fresh spinach. If you're following a keto diet, this pizza is a must-have for weekend nights.

19. Baba Ganoush

Eat this eggplant dip with celery for the perfect in-between meal nibble. Thanks to a cup of tahini, this dip will add fat and flavour to an otherwise simple snack.

20. Thai Beef Satay

Marinating the beef in this keto recipe infuses it with an impressive amount of flavour in just 15 minutes. While that happens, you can quickly mix together the peanut sauce and accompanying salad for this Asian-style weeknight meal.

CONCLUSION

The epidemic of obesity suffered by the world population today is mainly due to the high consumption of processed foods, which are rich in preservatives, which are nothing but sugars, sodium and its derivatives or similar. This triggers our body to accumulate excess fat and develop problems in the heart and almost all of our systems. But with the help of ketogenic diets and intermittent fasting, the problems have been solved.